GINA RIPPON

The Lost Girls of Autism

The Untold Story of Women on the Spectrum

AF664630

PAN BOOKS

First published 2025 by Seal Press,
an imprint of Hachette Book Group, Inc

First published in the UK 2025 by Macmillan
This paperback edition first published 2026 by Pan Books
an imprint of Pan Macmillan
The Smithson, 6 Briset Street, London EC1M 5NR
EU representative: Macmillan Publishers Ireland Ltd, 1st Floor,
The Liffey Trust Centre, 117–126 Sheriff Street Upper,
Dublin 1 D01 YC43
Associated companies throughout the world

ISBN 978-1-0350-1164-3

Copyright © Gina Rippon 2025

The right of Gina Rippon to be identified as the author of this work has been asserted in accordance with the Copyright, Designs and Patents Act 1988.

All rights reserved. No part of this publication may be reproduced, stored in a retrieval system, or transmitted, in any form, or by any means (including, without limitation, electronic, mechanical, photocopying, recording or otherwise) without the prior written permission of the publisher.

Pan Macmillan does not have any control over, or any responsibility for, any author or third-party websites (including, without limitation, URLs, emails and QR codes) referred to in or on this book.

3 5 7 9 8 6 4

A CIP catalogue record for this book is available from the British Library.

Print book interior design by Bart Dawson.

Printed and bound in the UK using 100% Renewable Electricity by CPI Group (UK) Ltd

FSC www.fsc.org
MIX
Paper | Supporting responsible forestry
FSC® C116313

This book is sold subject to the condition that it shall not, by way of trade or otherwise, be lent, hired out, or otherwise circulated without the publisher's prior consent in any form of binding or cover other than that in which it is published and without a similar condition including this condition being imposed on the subsequent purchaser. The publisher does not authorize the use or reproduction of any part of this book in any manner for the purpose of training artificial intelligence technologies or systems. The publisher expressly reserves this book from the Text and Data Mining exception in accordance with Article 4(3) of the European Union Digital Single Market Directive 2019/790.

Visit **www.panmacmillan.com** to read more about all our books and to buy them.

To Grunya Efimovna Sukhareva and her girls
(PL, IW, WP, LK, and NW),
To Virginia, Barbara, and Elaine,
To Elfriede and Margarete,
And to all of autism's other lost people, named
and unnamed, found or still lost,
in the hope that you will never be forgotten again

Many of the moments when my autism caused problems, or at least marked me out as different, were those moments when I had come up against some unspoken law about how a girl or woman should be, and failed to meet it.

—Joanne Limburg, *Letters to My Weird Sisters: On Autism and Feminism*

CONTENTS

PREFACE

WHY ME AND WHY THIS BOOK?

I SHOULD START WITH A CONFESSION. I HAVE BEEN PART OF the problem I am hoping this book will solve.

Over many years, both as a researcher and teacher, as well as something of a social justice warrior, I have eagerly absorbed publications about how the world has short-changed women, not just way back in history, but here, now, in the twenty-first century. These are powerful books about medicine's gender problem, for example, or about the damage caused by data bias in a world designed for men. I have even written one myself, appealing to anyone who would listen, not to be misled by damaging myths about sex differences in the brain.[1]

My 'day job' involved the use of state-of-the-art brain-imaging techniques to investigate what is officially termed autism spectrum disorder (ASD). The research group I worked with was engaged in meticulous explorations of autistic brains to see if there were ways of profiling the activity in such brains, to explain why their owners experience the world so differently. When talking about this outside my lab, many people would say something along the lines of 'Autism – that's a boy thing, right?' And I would trot out the 'party line' that autism was, indeed, much more common in boys, perhaps four or five times as much, and that, although there were autistic girls, they were 'pretty rare'. I was conscious of the fact that very few of the autistic individuals we were testing were female, which confirmed this impression.

My wake-up call came when I and a group of feminist neuroscientists I had also been working with were taken to task by various high-end media outlets for 'putting women's lives at risk'. We had written several critical commentaries about research into sex differences in the brain. We had pointed out that all too often the researchers had gone beyond what they had actually found, over-enthusiastically describing tiny differences in group average data as 'profound' or 'fundamental', or failing to point out the huge number of comparisons that showed no differences at all.

Our intended message had been that this research was so important that we must be careful to do it well and, as importantly, be cautious about how we wrote about it. This apparently was not what was heard. We were accused of advocating a ban on sex difference research – 'sex differences deniers' and 'feminazis' were some of the more publishable epithets hurled our way. Why was this putting women's lives at risk? Because, it was fervently pointed out, there were many brain-based physical and mental conditions where sex differences were clear, so it was vital that all research into such conditions assume that biological sex was exerting some kind of powerful effect on who did or didn't succumb, and research programmes must be designed accordingly. Top of the list for 'male' conditions were almost invariably Parkinson's disease and autism. We feminazis could not and should not ignore 'male-specific risk mechanisms' and 'female-specific protective mechanisms'.

And that is when I started to pay much more attention to what research should be telling us about sex differences in autism in general, and about sex differences in autistic brains in particular. Why were fewer females diagnosed as autistic? What had brain imagers found so far in comparing the brains of autistic females with those of autistic males? No spoiler alert, but, as you will see, what I found certainly startled me out of my own biased view of autism and made me ashamed of how much I had unthinkingly contributed to the disconcerting state of affairs in autism brain research.

WHAT IS IT LIKE TO BE YOU? PRETENDING TO BE NORMAL

I should also have been taking note of the powerful personal testimonies from autistic women that had been emerging, actually some time before we brain imagers started paying attention (or not!) to the issue of the male bias in autism science. Bravely laying bare the difficulties they had struggled with all their lives, they were providing the answer to the question that autism researchers so rarely seemed to ask – 'What is it like to be you?' Some described their miserable school years, relentlessly being teased and bullied. Some described their 'diagnosis bingo', being offered 'generalized anxiety disorder', 'attention deficit hyperactivity disorder', 'borderline personality disorder', 'eating disorder' before eventually arriving at autism, not uncommonly in the context of becoming the mother of an autistic child and spotting their own autism when working through the diagnostic checklist with their child's clinician. The quirky titles of their books often brilliantly summed up what life as an unrecognized autistic woman was like: *Odd Girl Out: An Autistic Woman in a Neurotypical World*; *Nerdy, Shy, and Socially Inappropriate: A User Guide to an Asperger Life*; *Autism in Heels: The Untold Story of a Female Life on the Spectrum*; and (one of my personal favourites) *I Overcame My Autism and All I Got Was This Lousy Anxiety Disorder*.

To be fair to the autism research community, there were several scientists who *had* woken up to the issues of autism in females. They were asking the 'What is it like to be you?' question, and had started to lay out a framework to show what it was that autism researchers had been missing. Sometimes these scientists were themselves autistic, thus making them uniquely qualified to ask (and answer) such questions. Their enquiries began to reveal why it was that autism in girls and women had been overlooked for so long – often rather shockingly identifying just how many barriers have blocked their path to the recognition they needed.

'Pretending to be normal', as well as being the title of one of the female autism books, sums up a key issue in this whole saga. There appears to be a powerful drive in some autistic individuals, many of them female, to do everything they can to disguise their difficulties, to 'hide in plain sight' or 'fly beneath the radar', as it has been described. Understandably, this did not really come to light until these 'Chameleons', as they have been dubbed, themselves revealed their undercover activities. This book will show just how important the discovery of this camouflaging behaviour has been to uncovering the mystery of the missing autistic females. It also underscores how important it is to talk to the people you are studying!

Bearing this in mind, and having decided to explore the shortfalls in autism science that had led to so many autistic women being misdiagnosed or missed altogether, I didn't start by diving back beneath my brain scanner. I realized I should talk to as many girls and women as I could, to get a better handle on what their experiences were like. I wanted to write about the science behind the stories, but I wanted to get the stories first.

This was the most fascinating part of this book's journey. Face to face or via Zoom, in people's homes, in research centres, and in schools, I talked for hours to late-diagnosed women, to teenagers, to parents, carers, and teachers of autistic girls, and to the autistic girls themselves. The youngest of my interviewees was ten, the oldest was seventy-two (and just diagnosed!). Almost to a fault, they were among the most thoughtful and self-aware people I have ever met.

I wanted to keep the conversations as open-ended as possible, so there was no strict questionnaire-type format. But I nearly always included a version of 'What kind of questions about your autism do you think brain scientists should be asking?' Common responses were along the lines of 'Why do I get so panicked when people change their plans?' or 'Why does the world make me so anxious?' 'Does my brain make my clothes feel scratchy?' came from one of the younger interviewees.

To get some insight into their lived experiences, I also asked various versions of the 'What is it like to be you?' question. The answers, across all ages, almost all spoke of various kinds of social difficulties. They referred to being bullied, or called weird, or being drawn into abusive relationships. To 'standing on the outside of life looking in', revealing the importance of what social psychologists call 'belongingness', which seemed so much more intense in some of the girls and women I talked to.

This 'outsider' theme has come up time and again in the conversations I have had with autistic people over the years, females in particular. I heard it so often from the people I spoke to for this book that I was tempted to incorporate 'through the looking glass' into its title (acknowledging, of course, that there was a precedent). I got quite carried away with this as a possible authorly device, which was partly why I have used the name Alice in the introduction to this book. As it turned out, my pleasingly original idea was not that original after all. Joanne Limburg, author of the wonderful autism book *Letters to My Weird Sisters*, has also published a book of poems called *The Autistic Alice*, which even has a cover that looks like a small child reaching through a mirror. And there is also a child's book called *Alice, an Autistic Aardvark*! So, nothing new under the sun then, but at least a confirmation that this outsider-ness is registered as part of the autistic experience.

There was also a certain amount of disquiet (to put it politely) at how hard it had been to get a diagnosis of autism for themselves or their daughters. This was not to do with long waiting lists for autism diagnoses; it was to do with getting past the 'autism is a boy thing' attitude when they asked for help. One of my interviewees had a son who had already been diagnosed with autism but was 'given the brush off' when she raised the possibility that her daughter might also be autistic. She was told that she was being hypersensitive about her daughter (who was eventually diagnosed as autistic at the age of twelve, having been referred to an eating disorder clinic by the special needs coordinator at her secondary school). So this book is also about the detective work behind diagnosing autism and why, until quite recently, it has failed to spot so many who needed to find their place on the spectrum.

I used the material from these interviews to determine what aspects of autism I would focus on, and, in a few cases, selected quotes from the interviewees who, as ever, made their points so much more tellingly than I could ever have done. (Look out for the brilliant description from one woman about her life as an untrained undercover agent.) I have not used the real names of the interviewees except in one or two specific cases, and I have made efforts to anonymize any stories that might identify any of my interviewees without their explicit consent.

I also managed to contact many of the researchers who have been responsible for finally sparking interest in autism in women. This was more to get insights into why and how they were asking the questions they did than to swap methodology tips. They were incredibly generous with their time, and helpfully willing to share their research stories. Any misrepresentation or misapprehension of their findings must be laid at my door and not theirs.

So, yes, girls do 'get' autism. You will find out that this was known for some time before the so-called 'fathers' of autism set out their stalls. You will find out how autism's male spotlight problem has skewed just about everything in the world of autism, from what it actually is and how it is measured, through to who is included in science's hunt to solve the autism puzzle. This book is the story of the lost girls of autism, and, hopefully, its telling will make sure they are afforded their rightful place on the spectrum.

SEX, GENDER, SEX/GENDER, GENDER/SEX

The terms *sex* and *gender* have become something of a hot topic in recent years, and it is important for readers to be clear how these terms are being used in this book. The World Health Organization (WHO) informs us that 'Sex refers to the biological characteristics that define humans as female or male. While these sets of biological characteristics are not mutually exclusive, as there are individuals who possess both, they tend to differentiate humans as males and females'.[2]

Broadly speaking, the relevant 'biological characteristics' can be grouped into genes, genitals, and gonads – measures of which have historically (and medically) been used to divide the human race into two categories, female and male, in accord with what the

WHO is telling us. When we speak of sex differences, therefore, we should normally be limiting ourselves to those aspects of the human condition that relate only to biological factors, such as chromosomes and hormones. In the past, however, the term *sex differences* has also been applied to additional human characteristics such as personality and temperament, or cognitive and emotional skills, with the assumption that these are causally linked to sex-differentiated biology. Further, social roles have been similarly linked to biology, accounting for differences in educational achievement, career choice, or leadership skills, for example. The underlying assumption was that who you were, and what you could do, was biologically determined, hardwired, fixed, inevitable, and invariant. This is known as the essentialist or 'nature' argument.

Such extreme essentialist arguments have been dismantled in recent years, with powerful evidence that much of the variability in humans is not solely determined by sex, but is also influenced by powerful, lifelong external factors such as education and socio-economic status, and by experiential differences that may well reflect different social and cultural opportunities.

'Gender', the WHO tells us, 'refers to the characteristics of women, men, girls and boys that are socially constructed. This includes norms, behaviours, and roles associated with being a woman, man, girl or boy, as well as relationships with each other. As a social construct, gender varies from society to society and can change over time'.[3]

Linked to the emerging feminist arguments in the 1970s and 80s, this social constructionist approach asserted that biology was broadly irrelevant in determining social roles and status, and that any evidence of social and cultural differences between females and males should be referred to as gender differences and linked to social construction or 'nurture'. However, over time, the term *gender* has come to be applied to all aspects of being female and male, including these very categories. Hence, gender pay gaps or, even worse, gender reveal parties.

In the twenty-first century, particularly in the light of contemporary understanding of how much our brains can be influenced by social pressures, it is becoming harder and harder to sustain a neat distinction between 'sex' and 'gender', between 'nature' and 'nurture'. Biology is not irrelevant in understanding psychological and social differences between females and males, but its influence is clearly powerfully moderated by external factors. As I have described elsewhere, we are looking at a biological script playing out on a social stage. This may well be as true in understanding autism as in understanding female/male differences in general.

In academic circles, the use of terms such as 'sex/gender' or 'gender/sex' has been offered as a solution to the evident entanglement of biology with society, of society with biology. This terminology flags up the need to acknowledge the likely influence of both in determining individual differences. Coming back to the WHO, we are told that 'Gender interacts with, but is different from, sex'.[4]

The starting point of much of the work I shall refer to in this book is an emphasis on the primary role of biology in discussions about autism in general, and in discussions about why there are apparently fewer females than males diagnosed as being on the spectrum. Hence, you will come across the terms 'sex' and 'sex differences' more frequently than 'gender' and 'gender differences'. But, as part of my argument is that socialization factors can be inextricably entangled with biological factors and both will have a powerful role to play in the different presentation of autism in girls and women, the term 'sex/gender' will also make an appearance.

GENDER IDENTITY

As we shall see, issues of autism and autism identity also intersect with those of gender identity, so some understanding of associated terminology will be needed. Going back to definitions from the WHO, we find that '"gender identity" refers to a person's deeply felt, internal and individual experience of gender, which may or may not correspond to the person's physiology or designated sex at birth.'[5] In the twenty-first century, the relationship between personal identity and biological characteristics associated with sex assigned at birth has become a matter of intense debate, often at odds with the WHO's cautious definition. In addition, there are challenges to the notion that gender identity can only be a binary choice between the categories of female and male, feminine and masculine, again as associated with biological sex.

The term *transgender* refers to individuals who feel their gender identity does not match the sex category to which they were assigned at birth, based on the presence of female or male genitalia. In some instances, such individuals may wish to be identified as of a different sex and/or gender. This is linked to the traditional binary understanding of female and male, with some individuals assigned female at birth transitioning to a male identity or some individuals assigned male at birth transitioning to a female identity. Transgender people might choose to dress and behave in ways more associated with a different gender, with multiple genders, or with androgyny. They may also choose to undertake medical procedures to alter bodily sexual characteristics.

Gender identity issues can also mark a move away from traditional binary female/male categories, with the term *gender diversity* encompassing a wide range of gender identities. The term can include transgender people, as above, but also non-binary individuals, who do not identify exclusively as male or female. Additionally, there are individuals whose gender identity may change over time or who reject the idea of a fixed gender altogether.

There is strong evidence of an intersection of autism and gender in issues of identity. There are reports of higher rates of gender diversity in autistic populations than in non-autistic populations, with one study finding that as many as 15 per cent of autistic adults identify as trans or non-binary, with higher rates among those identified as female at birth.[6] There are claims that autism, or high levels of autistic traits, is three to six times as common in transgender or gender variant populations.

Understanding this intersection of autism with gender identity may not only provide valuable insights into autism itself, but also offer a lens through which to view issues of personal identity.

Within discussions of gender identity and gender diversity, 'assigned female at birth' and 'assigned male at birth' are emerging as terms more acceptable to the gender diverse community than 'female' and 'male'. These will be used when referencing such discussions and their links to autism. Otherwise, the terms 'female' and 'male' will be used throughout the book.

In writing not only about autism, but also matters of sex and gender, as well as contending with historical material where little or no attention was given to the stigmatizing possibilities of labels applied to what was seen as 'abnormal' behaviour, I appreciate the need for caution in the terms I will be using. So I thought it worth flagging up that I am aware of some of the sensitivities attached to different words and phrases, and will do my best to address these appropriately. In addition, we should be aware that some words may have subtly different meanings when used in an academic science context as opposed to everyday use.

WHEN IS A DIFFERENCE NOT A DIFFERENCE?

Caution is needed in the use of the term 'difference' when discussing group comparisons, in this instance between females and males and/or autistic and non-autistic groups. In common parlance, 'different' can imply 'distinct' or reliably distinguishable. When referring to the outcome of statistical comparisons, this impression can be compounded by the use of terms such as 'significantly different'. With respect to the kind of measures of behaviour or cognitive skills, it is rarely the case in comparisons of groups of females and males that the two populations are, indeed, distinctly different. Data from each group will show a certain amount of variability, and, more importantly, there will be considerable overlap between the two groups. So although there may be an average difference at the group level, it will be so small as to be virtually meaningless. At odds with populist presentations of female/male differences such as the Mars/Venus genre, made famous (or notorious) by John Gray's best-selling self-help relationship book *Men Are from Mars, Women Are from Venus*, women and men are often much more similar than they are different.

Overall, when describing the results of research studies, I will use the term 'different' (or even 'significantly different') in its statistical sense, but would not want this taken to mean that the findings have proved the existence of two or more distinct groups.

DISORDERED, DYSFUNCTIONAL, OR JUST DIFFERENT?

The term for autism as used by official diagnostic manuals is currently 'autism spectrum disorder,' in line with the terminology for other mental health conditions such as depressive disorder. 'Disorder' implies a deviation from some objectively determined acceptable norm – perhaps the presence of some form of atypical (or 'abnormal') behaviour in the individual being studied would come into this category. The use of the term 'disorder' is firmly tied to the medical model of mental health problems, that there is some pathological process underlying an individual's unusual behaviour. The implication of terms such as 'disorder' and 'dysfunction' is that there is something wrong with an individual, something about her or him that needs correcting in order to bring them in line with the rest of the world.

Advocates for the autism community have drawn attention to the potentially stigmatizing use of the terms 'disorder' or 'deficit', particularly when they refer to patterns of behaviour that may readily be found in so-called 'typical' populations, but are perhaps expressed in more extreme forms by autistic people. Rigid adherence to routines is characteristic of many autistic people. This could be viewed as a strength, and accommodation could be made, for example, by ensuring that any changes to an autistic person's schedule were clearly flagged in advance. Similarly, adjustment to the environment, or to the stereotypical expectations found there, could normalize certain autistic behaviours. Motor stereotypes such as hand-flapping or finger-tapping are common in autistic populations. They have been identified as an adaptive or calming response to disturbing levels of sensory stimulation or to anxiety induced by an unexpectedly unpredictable environment. Yet, self-stimulation, or *stimming* as it is called, is often deemed socially unacceptable, and can be the subject of 're-education' programmes to train autistic individuals to eliminate or suppress such behaviour. But an alternative solution could be to accommodate stimming and accept it as part of an autistic individual's way of dealing with the world.

Issues such as these are part of the neurodiversity movement, which advocates that those with less usual ways of behaving should be accepted, accommodations should be made for them, and they should not be treated as in need of therapies or cures. As part of this approach, it is felt that the term 'disorder' should be avoided. To support this, 'autism spectrum disorder' should become 'autism spectrum condition'. 'Autism spectrum condition' can be found in more recent writings about autism, but most research papers, particularly in the field of neuroscience, still refer to autism spectrum disorder or ASD. Where I cover such work, the term ASD may therefore appear, but I will do my best to use the term 'condition' where possible.

However, in the context of the current concept of autism as a spectrum, it should be remembered that the term also encompasses individuals who display extremely challenging behaviours, may be nonverbal and self-injurious, and will require lifelong care. The terms 'disorder' and 'disability' may well be used more often by those researching or working with such communities. In addition, 'profound autism' has been proposed as a term to apply to those who require constant care and have limited or no language and significant intellectual disability.[7] We should acknowledge that this term has not been universally accepted within the autism community, but it is sometimes encountered in clinical or research categories and so is a term used in this book.[8]

The terms 'puzzle' and 'jigsaw' have often been used in the past as metaphors to convey the complexity of autism, but more recently have attracted some criticism. This is because they can be taken to imply that autism is something to be decoded or fixed, or is difficult to understand. When this matter was raised following a sensitivity read of this book, I contacted some of my interviewees for their opinions. None of them felt that such terms were disrespectful of the autistic experience, although (once I had raised it!) they could see how they might be thought problematic. Where possible, I have altered the use of such terms, but, occasionally, I have used them when reflecting the context in which they were originally employed.

In the same vein, terms such as 'risk', 'at risk', 'high risk', and 'vulnerability' have been criticized as equating autism with a pathological condition (possibly to be avoided). In many cases, these terms reflect specific scientific terminology; for example, when identifying genetic factors or selecting the siblings of autistic children for study on the basis of their increased possibility of also being autistic. It is in this sense that you will find these terms used in this book.

MATTERS OF IDENTITY

One aspect of the destigmatizing of autism is an emphasis on the condition as having a specific and positive identity. As a consequence, it is suggested that individuals with an autism diagnosis should be referred to as 'autistic people' (identity-first language) rather than 'people with autism' (person-first language), as the latter implies that autism should be considered as separate from who they are, and perhaps as somehow negative. I will generally use the former term, although the latter might come up in describing earlier coverage of the autism story.

Autism as an identity is also a clear theme in many of the personal testimonies of late-diagnosed autistic women, where a powerful aspect of the relief they report when diagnosed refers to finding their 'tribe', a recognizable community to which they belonged, where their lived experiences finally made sense. So one serious consequence of large numbers of people apparently being overlooked by the current diagnostic process is that, as well as being deprived of help and support, they may also be deprived of an identity. Therefore, in discussing matters linked to the 'what is autism?' question, it should be acknowledged that answers should cover more than diagnostic and scientific issues.

Having started this preface with a confession, I shall finish with an apology. The focus of this book comes very much from a WEIRD (Western, Educated, Industrial, Rich, and Democratic) perspective. This reflects my own experience and the research culture in which my career has been embedded. With respect to the wider social issues raised in this book, I must acknowledge, for example, that the intersecting experiences of being both female and a person of colour have not been covered. Sadly, this reflects the state of research to date, and hopefully will be addressed in the future. Should I have a chance to be academically reborn, I would love to be an anthropologist exploring autism issues in different cultures. I believe this would intersect powerfully with questions about gendered socialization, and could indeed shed some light on how cultural pressures determine the expression of autistic differences, and how these are perceived in different cultures. Autistic people of colour may be even more susceptible to those pressures of conformity and the fear of exclusion that I identify as relevant to the under-representation of women in autism. Sadly, the question of race and its impact on autism's presentation is outside the scope of this book, but it is clearly an area where further research is needed. I am sorry that I could not include it here, but hopefully the appropriate baton will be picked up soon.

Overall, I hope that no one finds any of the terminology used in this book insensitive or offensive. I asked many of the people I had interviewed to flag up any such problems (as if they hadn't already done enough for me!) and made changes where necessary. If there are any terms or comments that cause discomfort, I take full responsibility and will certainly avoid them in the future.

INTRODUCTION

If you google 'famous historical figures who might have been autistic,' the list of results will be headed by figures such as Albert Einstein, Thomas Jefferson, Nikola Tesla, and Hans Christian Andersen. If you ask someone to name famous people (fictional or real) who are known for having autism or being 'on the spectrum', Raymond Babbitt, the main character in the movie *Rain Man*, is often the favourite, possibly followed by Sherlock Holmes (especially in his recent incarnation by Benedict Cumberbatch) and Sheldon in *The Big Bang Theory*. No women will figure. There is a powerful popular conception of autism as a world of socially awkward, male creative geniuses whose divergent thinking may have driven human progress, but whose idea of small talk at a party might involve a monologue about steam trains. The individual presentations may differ but the common characteristic is that they will almost invariably be male.

This impression is backed up by repeated claims in research papers, on autism websites, and in autism advice manuals that boys are, on average, four times more likely to be diagnosed with autism than girls. (Spoiler alert – we should note that such statistics refer to the likelihood of *being diagnosed* with autism. As we shall see, that is not necessarily the same as 'having' autism.) This belief in the maleness of autism even informs the world of in vitro fertilization, where choosing a female embryo to avoid the possibility of autism can be part of pre-implantation gender selection advice in places like Australia. This, perhaps more than anything, indicates what a powerful hold the notion of autism as a boy thing has on our understanding of the condition.

According to the WHO, it is estimated that about 1 per cent of the world's population has ASD – over 75,000,000 people. And, again, the WHO reports that autism is nearly four times more common among boys than girls.[1] In 2023, the U.S. Centers for Disease Control and Prevention (CDC) reported that one in thirty-six children is diagnosed with an ASD.[2] In the UK it has been estimated as one in fifty-seven.[3] Again, it is worth noting the phrase 'is diagnosed with'. The confident reporting of such statistics carries the implication that there is a universally agreed measure of this particular condition, carefully constructed, with assured reliability and validity. It suggests that there is a well-established and long-standing database, with a range of norms and statistical measures, adjusted for variables such as age, gender, socio-economic status, level of education, different languages, different cultures. It suggests that autism is an easily recognized and readily described condition. A glimpse at the history of autism reveals that this has never really been the case.

The very first boy to be formally diagnosed as autistic, Donald Triplett, only died in June of 2023, at the age of eighty-nine. If you track descriptions of autism over the years since five-year-old Donald's diagnosis by the Austrian child psychiatrist Leo Kanner, its shape-shifting nature becomes clear. Initially described as 'rare', we are now apparently looking at prevalence rates of one in thirty-six. But this figure can vary from place to place, even clinic to clinic. Autism has been described as a stigmatizing condition, with autistic people historically being shunned and institutionalized, but it has also been hailed as a significant 'tribe' to which previously homeless, 'othered' individuals are thrilled to be admitted. This lack of clarity can affect everything from research agendas to educational care plans, from self-identity to cultural expectations and stereotypes. And, of course, it will be a factor in deciding who is or isn't autistic. But the consistent message has somehow always remained that autism, whatever it actually is, is more common among boys.

But, in the last decade or so, there has been a wave of powerful personal testimonies from late-diagnosed autistic women who had not been 'spotted' until their thirties, forties, fifties, or even later. In the first decade of this century, there were a number of books published by such women, writing about their lifelong struggles with feeling different or weird (or being treated as such) – with not fitting in, with finding themselves in inappropriate and/or abusive relationships, with having a feeling that they were always on the outside looking in, as I described in the preface. Some of the titles tell it all: *Pretending to Be Normal* by Liane Willey, *Odd Girl Out* by Laura James, *Nerdy, Shy, and Socially Inappropriate* by Cynthia Kim, and *Autism in Heels: The Untold Story of a Female Life on the Spectrum* by Jennifer Cooke O'Toole. Not only were these women demonstrating that there were, indeed, women out there with autism, but they were spelling out, loudly and clearly, what it was like to be autistic, to experience the world differently, to live a different kind of life.

They have always been there. Why have we missed them?

The absence of women from the autism story is not because it actually *is* a story that can only be about men and boys, but because no one had ever challenged this stereotype. The dawning awareness of this 'male spotlight' problem has impacted all parts of the autism community and is starting to uncover its downstream consequences. We find that clinicians have refused referrals because 'women don't get autism' or because they didn't appear to fit the male-based stereotype of friendless loners who avoid eye contact. We hear stories of parents, even those with sons who had already been diagnosed with autism, having to exaggerate their daughter's struggles to get the help she needed. Scientists are waking up to the fact that all their research to date has been skewed by the lack of female participants, screened out by the rigid, male-based criteria of the so-called gold standard autism assessment schedules. And there are too many stories of women who have suffered decades of mislabelled and mistreated mental health problems before someone said, 'I wonder if you might be autistic'.

Why should it matter that women had been overlooked in the unfolding story of autism? Because it means that, in our search for an understanding of autism, our search area has been too narrow – diagnostic dice have been loaded, clinical decisions have been distorted, research agendas have been constrained, and autism awareness programmes have been limited. The model of autism as a 'boy thing' has affected our efforts to find out its causes, to understand the lived experiences of *all* of those who are autistic, to identify the most effective support. And there may indeed be parallels with other stories where women have been overlooked or ignored, as chronicled in, for example, Caroline Criado Perez's *Invisible Women: Data Bias in a World Designed for Men*, or Elinor Cleghorn's *Unwell Women: A Journey through Medicine and Myth in a Man-Made World*.

It turns out that the idea of autism as a male problem might actually be a form of self-fulfilling prophecy. If clinicians meet a young boy with disturbed patterns of behaviour and delayed cognitive and social development, they are much more likely to reach for their autism screening schedules than if they encounter a girl with similar characteristics. Even if such clinicians do ignore the odds and look for autism in their girl referrals, it has been shown that the diagnostic tools they use can actively screen out girls, as they have been developed by focussing on problems in boys. Girls with behavioural problems are much more likely to be given alternative diagnoses such as social anxiety or borderline personality disorder, so they don't figure in the autism statistics. Others who might be well-placed to spot those who are having daily struggles can be blinkered by beliefs in autism as a male problem. I have met teachers who have told me that in their thirty years of teaching they have never encountered an autistic girl. A recent study showed that teachers given identical scenarios of problematic behaviour were much more likely to conclude that the child might be autistic (and would need help) if they were told that it was a boy.[4]

How has this affected people like me, a research scientist who has studied autism for decades? If a key characteristic of the condition is its maleness, then it is this aspect of human biology that will primarily determine the focus of the research we carry out, the variables we measure, the cohorts we recruit. Geneticists will root around on X chromosomes to see if they can discover the source of the 'female protective effect'. Endocrinologists will explore the effects of testosterone on behaviour in order to understand a 'male vulnerability factor'. Brain scientists will research links between 'male brains' and autism. Researchers will only recruit their participants from among those with an official diagnosis of autism, and will build their models of autism's characteristics and causes from this skewed community, the male one.

It is becoming increasingly evident that over many decades of research, we have actually excluded, overlooked, or ignored a significant proportion of people who present with the very condition we are looking at. As a result, the carefully thought out research programmes we have been putting together, the next round of tests we want to try out, the tentative explanations we are proposing, could be misinformed and potentially misleading.

AUTISM'S MISSING GIRLS: WHERE HAVE THEY BEEN?

In order to unpick this puzzle, it is important to start at the beginning. How did the emergence and evolution of the condition we now refer to as autism, which allegedly affects one in thirty-six people today, come to, at best, underestimate or, at worst, overlook, so many additional members of their community? From the outset, it has been clear that women *can* be autistic – in the most well-known early description of autism, a 1943 report by Leo Kanner, three girls were described in addition to eight boys.[5] But the 'maleness' of the condition was established sufficiently early in autism's timeline that it became a self-fulfilling prophecy, with this belief guiding diagnostic decisions and slowly, but surely, increasing the male:female ratio in diagnosed autistic populations.

As long ago as the 1980s, there were some early discussions about autism's missing females in the clinical and academic literature. The UK psychiatrist and researcher Lorna Wing, one of the key players in the widening of diagnostic criteria and the development of our modern-day understanding of autism, commented at that time on the lower numbers of females in the reported statistics.[6] She (presciently) speculated that perhaps females were better at disguising their difficulties; so there might be more autistic women than had been counted, but they were hiding in plain sight, or flying beneath the diagnostic radar.

Others suggested that autistic females presented with a 'milder' form of autism, so did not pass the diagnostic threshold. There seemed to be no discussion that this might have something to do with the threshold itself. The definitive maleness of autism seemed to be a given – there was little suggestion that the system for recognizing autism may be at fault and that the male:female ratios were reflecting a flawed system.

It was really the voices of autistic women themselves, and those insightful researchers who listened to them, that shook up the world of autism. As well as the autobiographies mentioned previously, autistic women harnessed the power of social media with YouTube videos such as Hannah Belcher's *Changing the Face of Autism: Here Come the Girls* and Barb Cook's *The Chameleons: Women with Autism Spectrum Disorder*. In 2015, the British television network ITV aired the documentary *Girls with Autism*, about Limpsfield Grange School in Surrey, a state-funded residential special school for girls with communication and social interaction difficulties, including autism. In 2017, the research journal *Autism* published an entire special issue titled 'Women and Girls on the Autism Spectrum'. The website Autistic Girls Network, campaigning for better recognition and diagnosis of autistic girls and non-binary young people, was launched the same year. People were starting to pay attention.

Some researchers suggested that perhaps autism had been overlooked in women because it presented differently. An ever-changing array of diagnostic manuals had focussed on the presentation of autism in those in whom it was most commonly spotted – the boys. So, in another of those self-fulfilling prophecies that seem to characterize this particular narrative, if you were a girl and didn't behave like an autistic boy, then it was assumed you weren't autistic. This might seem like an admirably 'gender-free' or 'gender-irrelevant' approach to diagnosis, but it does presume that, in fact, gender *is* irrelevant. And you could only determine whether or not gender *was* irrelevant by checking to see if the manifestation of female autism (or phenotype) was different from the male autism one. Up until the early 2000s, little attention had been paid to whether diagnosed females were markedly different from diagnosed males. Given the male bias in the diagnostic schedules being used, those females who did 'make the cut' were, of course, quite likely to be pretty similar to diagnosed males. So there needed to be more of a focus on the possibility that autism might present differently in females.

So, researchers started listening to the people they were researching. They went beyond just devising complicated tasks that were supposed to measure the difficulties that previous researchers had concluded were the defining characteristics of autism. It became clear that for many diagnosed women, or women with high levels of autistic traits, the need to fit in, to have friends, to avoid being noticed as different, was a powerful driving force in how they interacted with other people – much more so than for autistic males. Take Gill, one of the late-diagnosed females who shared her story with me, who still remembers the pain of realizing that she had always been overlooked by her contemporaries:

> I still remember the moment when I realized I really didn't fit in. The school had a big thing about class photos in your last year, and we all got to get copies and get them signed by everybody so we would remember all of our school friends forever. So you really had to be there and groups of special friends made arrangements with each other to make sure they stood together. I got the time wrong and missed the photo shoot. No one came looking for me because no one noticed I wasn't there. So, in that

'precious' memento of my time at school, I am nowhere to be seen. Which pretty much says it all.

Worrying about fitting in was, of course, at odds with the classic aloof loner image of autism and certainly wasn't the kind of behaviour that, up to that point, was being studied by brain scanners or via questionnaires. Once researchers started to focus on autistic women's lived experiences, it turned out they could identify common themes. This meant they could then generate self-report questionnaires that tapped into the realities of everyday life for autistic females and could quantify key aspects of their experiences across groups of participants. We were, at last, starting to build a picture of what it was like to be female and to be autistic.

'YOU MUST BECOME A CHAMELEON TO SURVIVE'

One consistent theme that runs through both the personal testimonies and the research findings is that so-called camouflaging or masking is a pattern of behaviour that is more common in autistic women than in autistic men. We will return to this theme throughout this book. Masking includes a range of strategies employed to disguise autistic traits, or to 'pass' as normal. It can include training yourself to maintain eye contact, or mimicking gestures and body language, even devising and rehearsing elaborate social scripts in advance of social events. This pattern has become a key focus of much of the contemporary research into sex differences in autism. On the surface, being able to disguise your difficulties sufficiently to 'pass as normal' might seem like an adaptive strategy, especially as 'fitting in' is such a powerful social drive. There is also evidence, especially from observational studies and personal testimonies, that even very young girls display these kinds of behaviour, which could partly explain findings showing that girls are diagnosed at least two years later than boys, and that it takes longer to get a diagnosis for girls once concerns have been expressed.

But there is a dark side to camouflaging behaviour, again only becoming clear once autistic women were asked to share their experiences. The daily effort of monitoring and adjusting behaviour to fit in can be mentally exhausting and lead to heightened stress and anxiety, eventually even collapse and burnout. Maintaining a façade can cause identity issues, with the constantly changing masks hiding an individual's true self and, paradoxically, preventing genuine relationships. The loss of self-esteem and feelings of inadequacy associated with repeated failures to fit in can lead to depression and even suicide. So understanding the motivation behind this high-risk social strategy is key to gaining new insights into autism, especially as it more commonly presents in women.

This newer perspective on aspects of autism in females raises wider issues. Why might camouflaging be more common among autistic females? Is it due to a particular characteristic of autism more common in females, or is it, more fundamentally, a particular characteristic more common in *all* females? Discussing sex/gender differences in autism has strong parallels with contemporary discussions about sex/gender differences in the wider population. Age-old discussions have taken place about the different demands that the world makes on females as opposed to males and, indeed, how females respond to these demands. Is the need to belong more powerful in females? Do females have some kind of innate social awareness that gives them a head start in social situations? Or are we looking at the consequences of sex-based biases in social programming? Do girls face more pressure to play nicely together, stay quiet, and obey the rules? As is so often the case, the atypical world can offer powerful insights into what is going on in 'everyday' life.

The study of camouflaging behaviour in autistic women is driving the new agenda in autism research. This is a pattern of behaviour that seems to set this particular group apart. They appear to be highly socially motivated to fit in, to belong, which is at odds with the traditional picture of autism. But the strategies women adopt to achieve this belonging appear to be only partially effective, if at all, and are also mentally and physically damaging. Yet still they persist. What is it that drives these individuals to put themselves through this day after day?

Part of the answer, at least, may lie in our newer understanding of the brain's role in making sure we humans are socially accepted and well embedded in our social networks. The human brain does not just provide the foundation of individual human abilities such as language or abstract thought or artistic and scientific creativity. It also, perhaps more significantly, ensures our survival and success as social beings, as individuals who will fit in with others. We have a powerful need to interact with others, and our behaviour is constantly adapted to fulfil that need. And this need appears to be a fundamental human driver. Group acceptance will provide a powerful reward, whereas social rejection or ostracism will be a devastating experience and should be avoided at all costs.

Brain imagers can demonstrate the effects that social interactions (or lack of them) have on the human brain and human behaviour. The brain networks activated by social rejection are the same networks activated by real physical pain – so not belonging or not fitting in is a powerfully aversive experience. The networks activated are also associated with severe mental health problems such as self-harm and eating disorders, disorders with the highest mortality rates of all. So fitting in and avoiding ostracism can, for some of us at least, be more than a social nicety and feel more like a matter of life or death.

Autistic individuals may withdraw from a world that brings such pain. Or they might painstakingly develop a set of strategies and elaborate social scripts that allow them to be accepted and included by those around them. As time goes on, the costs of these camouflaging or masking behaviours build up, but they persist, because fitting in, and not being dismissed as weird, is more important than anything else.

This drive for social acceptance can provide a new filter through which we can explore the autistic brain. A focus on the structures and functions of the social brain, with particular attention to the patterns of activation associated with the social reward system, could have a better chance at revealing more answers about autism.

For research scientists like me, the dawning awareness that autism in females might be different from autism in males was a wake-up call. Decades of research would need to be revisited to see if the conclusions we had confidently (or even tentatively) reached actually applied to only part of the autism community. If there were aspects of autism that were different in females, then we would need to replicate the work previously carried out only with males to see if we came up with the same answers when we included females. If the questions we were asking were based on assumptions that were true of only part of the autistic population, then we would need to ask different questions. If we had a fixed picture of reduced social activity in our autistic participants (because that was what the diagnostic schedules were telling us), and it turned out that there was a pattern of behaviour that indicated obsessively *over*active social behaviour in an overlooked group of our autistic participants, then a rethink was definitely called for.

The new 'vision' of female autism needs to inform more than the research world. Many late-diagnosed women have run the full gamut of alternative labels for their distress, with associated ineffective treatments and therapies. Autism is a lifelong condition, present from birth, so if you are not diagnosed until you are in your thirties or forties or fifties, or even older, you may well have suffered decades of misery and misunderstanding. Once you do get recognized, you will find that all the support is geared towards young children. You will have to confront the disbelief of others that you can't be autistic because you don't conform to the stereotype of a nerdy, male loner. At every level, the current unbalanced picture of autism is causing multiple problems for a significant number of women and girls who badly need help. We need to put this right.

Bringing females into the fold of the autistic community is about more than completing a membership checklist. One of the responses most often reported by women on receiving a (late) diagnosis of autism is of overwhelming relief, of 'finding their tribe'. At last, they have received an explanation for a life of being 'othered', of being labelled as 'weird,' of always feeling as if they were an outsider. Of trying so hard to be like other people that they lost a sense of their own identity, of continually (and mainly unsuccessfully) 'pretending to be normal', of suffering inexplicable bouts of mental illness and of being offered virtually all available diagnostic labels except the one that finally made sense, that of autism.

Given the powerful human need to belong, a positive self-identity brings a sense of well-being and boosts self-esteem. Whatever the rights and wrongs of the labels we humans attach to others, and ourselves, they do serve a purpose. They can give us a sense of self, offer some kind of explanation and expectation of what we are like, how we will behave, how we might get things wrong. If we are deprived of such a label, or are given the wrong one, it can have profound influences on our self-identity, our self-esteem, our social acceptance or rejection. Therefore, with respect to autism, it is important that we have a clear-eyed view of what it means to be autistic and especially why it might be different for different people, both female and male.

ALICE'S STORY

Let me introduce you to Alice, whose story typifies many of the struggles autistic women have faced. Alice is not her real name, and her story represents and reflects several of the lived experiences that autistic women shared with me when I was preparing this book, some of whom wished to be heard but not named. As explained in the preface, I have been struck by the similarities between the tales of life as an undiagnosed autistic woman I was hearing from my interviewees, and the adventures of Lewis Carroll's Alice, in both *Alice in Wonderland* and *Through the Looking-Glass*. So I chose the name Alice to represent these women. Alice was a mature student with two young sons, the elder severely autistic, his younger brother neurotypical. Alice had had many mental health struggles during her time at university. After nearly three years of pleading for an autism assessment, it was eventually confirmed that she was indeed on the spectrum and clearly always had been.

Over the years she had received many different diagnoses – the most recent was borderline personality disorder with social anxiety. It was not until what she called her 'light bulb moment' that she started the quest to 'prove' she was on the autistic spectrum.

The light bulb moment came when she accompanied her second child, Peter, aged two and a half, to his first day at nursery school. Alice had had a miserable time in her own school years, especially in secondary school, and had eventually become a school refuser. Her first son had never made it to any kind of mainstream schooling, so she was anxious to see how Peter would settle into his 'normal' nursery. She had visited the nursery on several occasions and had walked Peter there to make sure he would not be anxious about this new experience. She had asked to stay for his first morning at least to make sure he settled.

As soon as they arrived, Peter dived into the melee of early morning nursery, pausing only to hang his coat on the peg as Alice had made him practise at home. Stunned, Alice watched her tiny son effortlessly fit into what seemed to her to be a maelstrom of potential social pitfalls.

> He was a native of the world I had been watching from the outside all my life. Nobody had to tell him how to fit into the group around the sandpit. He cheerily handed over the toy saucepan he'd picked out of the toy box to the girls constructing a kitchen, who then included him in their activities. He roared around the playground playing some kind of game with apparently rigid but invisible rules. He just seemed to automatically . . . belong. I suddenly realized that I was looking at what *not* being autistic meant. I knew then that he had all the skills I had been missing. I knew then that I was autistic.

A nursery worker, watching Alice's anxious scrutiny, came over. 'Looks like he's having a good time', she said reassuringly. Alice could only ask: 'How does he know how to do that?!'

THIS BOOK IS ABOUT ALICE'S STORY, AND THE STORIES OF ALL the other Alices, misdiagnosed or missed altogether, and their invisible struggles with feeling 'other', their faces pressed against the window into a world to which they desperately wanted to belong.

Of the little Alices who painstakingly pieced together exquisitely detailed scripts they could follow to give them a role in that world, carefully camouflaging themselves to avoid being spotted as 'different'.

Of the teenage Alices, who became overwhelmed when their scripts were no longer fit for purpose, their world becoming too complicated and too exhausting to negotiate any more, with every day ending in meltdowns and tantrums, their distress expressing itself in ways that have attracted misleading labels – self-harm, eating disorders, gender dysphoria – masking their true problems.

And of the older Alices, some struggling through years of misunderstanding, mislabelling, and misguided treatment, many still standing on the other side of that looking glass, still 'othered', still exhausted by negotiating a social world through which everyone else seemed to sail through with automatic ease.

THIS BOOK IS IN TWO PARTS. THE FIRST WILL TAKE US BACK IN time to find out how and why clinicians and psychologists lost our autistic sisters in the first place. It explores how a persistent belief emerged that autism was primarily a condition found in boys, and how this belief skewed the early understanding of what autism looked like, and how it should be tested for. It then charts how powerful wake-up calls from these undetected women, as well as observant researchers, galvanized the autism world (and beyond) to start filling in the missing pieces of this part of the quest to understand autism. At last, we are starting to get a glimpse of an overlooked part of the autism spectrum.

The second part of the book investigates how this male spotlight has affected my world, the world of the autistic brain, and how scientists have also ignored autism's lost girls. You will see how the early years of autism brain research left females out of the equation altogether. Exciting developments in our understanding of the typical brain were enthusiastically adopted by autism researchers, but were only tested on the brains of autistic males. Luckily, the wake-up calls reached the research community as well, and we will see how brain scientists are finally beginning to unearth the neural underpinnings of this once hidden form of autism.

There is much more work to be done but we are starting to rebuild our picture of autistic behaviour and autistic brains, and as a bonus, gaining more understanding of human brains and human behaviour, to the benefit of us all.

PART I

HIDING IN PLAIN SIGHT

CHAPTER 1

WHAT IS AUTISM?

THE HUMPTY DUMPTY PROBLEM

When trying to answer what appears to be a straightforward question – what is autism? – we immediately encounter the amorphous nature of the definition of autism. If we had asked this question in the 1940s, we would have been given a different answer than if we had asked it in the 1980s, and we will see that the answer has changed yet again during the first two decades of this century. Echoing Alice's concern, we will discover that the term has been applied to an ever-widening collection of unusual behaviours, themselves packaged in a variety of different ways. It was originally used to describe a quite specific and rare type of behaviour, found in perhaps two to four cases per ten thousand children, but it has now become an umbrella term that is applied to a wide range of different behavioural problems, of different levels of severity, variously estimated to affect about one in a hundred children worldwide. It is also a term that has entered the public consciousness and so has acquired an even wider set of meanings and connotations.[1]

I was explaining these changes to the parents of a young autistic girl who had volunteered to speak to me as part of my information-gathering for this book. They had been offered many different suggestions as to what particular label her 'condition' should be given before 'autism' was finally settled on. Her father said he thought there was an element of shape-shifting in the terms he found in the many psychology and psychiatry textbooks he and his wife had pored over in their own search for an answer. His observation reminded me of a passage from Lewis Carroll's *Through the Looking-Glass*, which I borrowed for the subtitle of this chapter:

> 'When I use a word,' Humpty Dumpty said in rather a scornful tone, 'it means just what I choose it to mean – neither more nor less.' 'The question is,' said Alice, 'whether you can make words mean so many different things.'[2]

The origins of the word 'autism' are from the Greek word *autos*, meaning 'self'. The term was first used by the German psychiatrist Eugen Bleuler in 1911 to describe the kind of 'withdrawal into the self', or inward focus, that he felt was characteristic of the adult psychiatric patients he was studying. He believed that the delusions and hallucinations they reported might be linked to some kind of inner fantasy life that had somehow become an alternative reality.[3]

We now think of autism as primarily reflecting difficulties with understanding the outside world rather than the consequences of withdrawal into an inner one. The autistic inner world may be rich and complex but reflects the workings of an atypical literal mind often at odds with the inner worlds of others.

Post Bleuler, we find the term being applied to children whose many behavioural problems were associated with a marked lack of social engagement or 'aloofness', present from very early childhood. This became the defining characteristic of highly detailed individual case studies that were gradually being grouped together in order to be identified as a single syndrome. History has it that this cataloguing began with the work of Leo Kanner, who coined the term 'early infantile autism'.

The term continued to be used in the 40s and early 50s, applied to children whose primary characteristic seemed to be that they were 'living in a world of their own'. Early psychoanalytical approaches (falsely) linked this behaviour to some kind of traumatic maternal rejection causing a withdrawal from the outside world.[4] It became clear that the self-isolation that was evident in the early cases (whatever its cause) was a lifelong pattern of behaviour. Although there were other atypical characteristics, such as a rigid insistence on sameness in everyday routines, or persistent tic-like bodily movements, or obsessive fascination with obscure sets of information such as dates or weather patterns, the apparently implacable social withdrawal remained the main focus of clinicians and diagnosticians, and so the term 'autism' continued to be the defining label.

This association with isolation is reflected in the names for autism across the world. It is known as *zì bì zhèng* ('the lonely disease') in China, in Korea *chapae* ('closed in on oneself'), in Japanese *jheisyo* ('intentionally shut'), in Maori *takiwātanga* ('in their own time and space'). The Taiwanese version, *Xīngxīng -de háizi,* is more enigmatic and, rather beautifully, translates as 'children of the stars', unmindful of the outside world.

In autism research and advocacy circles, the public perception of autism and the growth of various stereotypes is often traced back to the film *Rain Man*, released in 1988. It starred Dustin Hoffman portraying an autistic man called Raymond Babbitt, who had amazing memory and mathematical abilities, but who also presented with severely impaired social behaviour. The presence of extraordinary skills, usually in domains such as art or music or memory or mathematics, is a very rare characteristic in autistic people, but it was this aspect of Raymond's autism that captured the public imagination and established another meaning for autism. The term 'a bit autistic' or 'a touch of autism' became more widely used in everyday conversation, suggesting the general population had a feeling that they knew what it meant. Hollywood-type coverage has left our society with the misguided and stereotypical idea of the autistic savant, with an amazing memory, astonishing mathematical or musical skills, or remarkable drawing abilities. The default autist is commonly conceived as a white, nerdy male who is enormously successful at anything to do with computers but has no social skills to speak of. You have to search long and hard to find a non-white autistic character in popular culture; Billy Cranston, the Blue Ranger in the 2017 *Power Rangers* film, being an unusual exception. You rarely see an autistic female in popular culture, though my contacts have mentioned Matilda from the television series *Everything's Gonna Be OK*. Saga Norén, the detective in the Scandinavian TV crime drama *The Bridge*, has widely been identified by viewers as on the spectrum, although not intentionally or explicitly identified as such. We might add Elizabeth Zott, the heroine of Bonnie Garmus's *Lessons in Chemistry*, to the list, although you might spot that she actually personifies typically male autistic characteristics. Paradoxically, it is also rare to see a child, given that autism is firmly labelled as a developmental disorder, present from birth, and that most diagnostic and therapeutic tools for autism are geared squarely towards children.

Looking at the rather flexible use of the term 'autism', then, does not really allow us to pin it down. Its definition will also vary depending on whom you ask. Clinicians will define autism as a clinical category, based on observation of behavioural patterns, with scores above or below a clinical threshold derived from diagnostic manuals or autism checklists. Geneticists may focus on narrow aspects of autistic behaviour in order to link them to genomes, whereas neuroscientists base their understanding on atypical patterns of brain connectivity and/or social brain networks. Psychologists experience patients exhibiting hyper-focus on local detail, or who are terrified of any break in routine. Parents will recount missed developmental milestones or daily struggles with the colours of food or the scratchiness of clothing labels, or in more severe cases, their experiences with a nonverbal, institutionalized child. More recently, autistic people themselves have found their voice, and speak of lifelong struggles to understand the invisible rules of being social, and the pain of social rejection or ostracism. Can the word 'autism' mean so many different things?

Perhaps if we return to those who first wrote about autism, we might gain some helpful insights.

THE 'FATHER(S) OF AUTISM'

In most writings about autism, including academic research papers, advice and advocacy websites, Leo Kanner, the Austrian-born psychiatrist who worked at Johns Hopkins Hospital in Baltimore, is known as the 'father of autism'. It is firmly asserted that the condition was first revealed by him in his 1943 paper 'Autistic Disturbances of Affective Contact'.[5] He described eleven children, eight boys and three girls, who showed severe behavioural impairments, with little or no language, or unfamiliar speech patterns and bodily movements such as hand-flapping or rocking or an unusual walking gait. Some children were set apart by highly restricted and hyper-focussed interests. All had an obsession with 'sameness' and became highly distressed by any departure from routine or by interruptions in the highly obsessive rituals they developed. For Kanner, the most striking impression was of the 'profound aloneness' and 'aloofness' of the children he studied. They appeared to have little or no wish for any kind of social engagement, and failed to respond to social overtures from others, even their parents. They appeared to be unaware of social rules.

Kanner was not the only clinician observing this self-isolating behaviour. It later emerged, in the 1980s, that another clinician, Hans Asperger, working in Vienna, had published a German language paper entitled 'Autistic Psychopathy in Childhood' in 1944, just a year after Kanner's paper was published.[6] Asperger described four boys in detail, although he had many previous years of clinical experience with children, both boys and girls, with various types of intellectual and behavioural impairments. Asperger also emphasized the lack of typical social engagement shown by the boys – 'severe difficulties of social integration'. Hence the term 'autistic' as used by both clinicians. But he also referred to high levels of original thought and special achievements, such as extraordinary calculating abilities. He has been credited with coining the term 'little professors' to refer to his boys. In describing one of them, Fritz V., Asperger comments that 'It is possible to consider such individuals both as child prodigies and as imbeciles, with ample justification'. Although Asperger's boys also displayed difficulties with language use, it was less to do with poor language or delayed language development, of the kind that went along with intellectual impairment of some kind, and more to do with unusual and apparently advanced ways of using language. For example, eight-year-old Harro described the difference between stairs and a ladder thus: 'Stairs are made out of stone. One doesn't call them rungs, they are called steps, because they are much bigger, and on the ladder they are thinner and smaller and round.'

Neither Kanner nor Asperger acknowledged each other's work, and it was assumed they had come up with the idea of autism independently. For the first thirty years or so of the study of autism, English-speaking researchers and clinicians were unaware of Asperger's work and the focus was on the identification and treatment of children suffering from 'Kanner's syndrome'. Diagnoses were still based on detailed case study reports from individual clinicians.

But as the number of cases increased and their details were collected together, the emerging image of autism was not clear-cut. The focus was still on the self-isolation and obsession with sameness identified by Kanner as the core elements of early childhood autism. However, there were many other inconsistent additions and observations, often a reflection of the beliefs of the clinician describing the children, and what they expected to see. This added up to a rather fuzzy picture of what autism actually was. Some clinicians focussed on the presence or absence of language, and any children who showed some form of speech development were excluded. Similarly, it was assumed that those who didn't display marked movement abnormalities such as rocking or hand-flapping couldn't be autistic.

Although both Kanner and Asperger focussed on autistic-like difficulties in social interaction, the case studies of children they wrote about paint rather different pictures. As we saw previously, Kanner's children seem to have been more severely impaired, with evidence of intellectual disability and language delays, whereas Asperger's boys seem less severely affected, with intact language development (if occasionally strange usage) and evidence of specialized skills (again in strangely narrow topics). We may be getting a picture of autistic behaviour, but we still seem some way from what the condition called autism actually is.

Perhaps studying the emergence of elaborate diagnostic schedules, backed up by weighty medical tomes, to be used by highly trained professionals might offer some kind of insight. Tracking the changes in how autism has been formally described over the years might reveal that, underneath all these changes, there *is* some kind of specific, distinct condition that clinicians and researchers were getting better at recognizing. The evolution of different diagnostic schedules to measure autism could reflect an increasingly better understanding of a condition that appeared to be slowly becoming more well-defined and more easily recognizable.

DIAGNOSING MENTAL HEALTH PROBLEMS

The evolution of a formal diagnosis of any psychiatric condition involves identifying common factors in available case histories and grouping them under a specific heading. These factors can then be assumed to be necessary to reliably diagnose a unique condition, possibly named after the discoverer – hence Kanner's syndrome and Asperger's syndrome. Once there is an agreed-upon set of diagnostic criteria, it should then be possible to investigate, for example, changes over time, the success or failure of different treatments, and the origins of the condition. The aim of developing this kind of classification system was modelled on the success of a similar cataloguing approach for physical illnesses; finding the symptoms that would help tell pneumonia and congestive heart failure apart, for example, had major implications for treatment and prognosis. Indeed, much of the history of psychiatry is a search for the physical bases of mental illnesses, which would mean that they could, rather paradoxically, no longer be counted as psychiatric conditions, but could be moved onto a list of illnesses with known physical origins. The history of syphilis, for example, showed that a physical source (a bacterium) could be the cause of insanity or madness, hence 'general paresis of the insane' disappeared to be replaced by the neurological disorder 'neurosyphilis'.

However, the psychiatric problems we are familiar with, such as depression and schizophrenia, as well as autism, do not have any easily measurable physical identifiers that are typical of that condition and (ideally) of no other. There are no physical characteristics, or biomarkers, that accompany unusual cognitive or behavioural patterns, no blood tests, brain scans, genome sequencing, hormonal assays, that anyone can use to reliably confirm that 'yes', this person is 'on the spectrum', they 'have' autism or they are 'autistic'.

So, instead, psychiatry had to fall back on what was really an elaborate extension of the early case study approach and generate a catalogue of 'standardised diagnostic criteria', an agreed-upon list of behavioural signs or symptoms that could be grouped together under a similarly agreed-upon diagnostic label. In the United States, the first example of such a catalogue, the *Statistical Manual of the Use of Institutions for the Insane* (SMUII), emerged in the 1920s, listing twenty-one disorders – almost all the more dramatic psychotic disorders, such as paranoia or paranoiac conditions, but also disorders with presciently vague and outdated names that jar against modern ears such as 'undiagnosed psychoses' or 'not insane'.[7]

It turned out that the notion of 'agreed-upon' and 'standardized' was more of a wish than a reality. Despite the emergence of another ten editions of SMUII and, later in the 1950s and 1960s, additional diagnostic manuals published by professional psychiatry associations, a survey in the 1970s showed that the hoped-for clarity and reliability of the increasing number of different conditions had never been achieved.[8] For example, it was reported that patients with exactly the same symptoms would be diagnosed with schizophrenia if they lived in New York, but manic-depressive disorder if they lived in London, which gives a clue as to how ill-defined each condition was.

International collaboration has improved the situation and each revision of the impressive tomes that now inform psychiatric diagnoses is the product of several years of deliberation by international experts. The fifth edition of the American Psychiatric Association's *Diagnostic and Statistical Manual of Mental Disorders* (DSM-5) is several inches thick and weighs in at approximately one thousand pages.[9] It includes over one hundred different overarching categories such as depressive disorders, disruptive impulse control disorders, and personality disorders, with dozens of subtypes linked to the nature and severity of the symptoms, the length of time they have been present, and the extent of distress they are causing. With such a volume, you would think we must have nailed down the explanations, can finely differentiate one form of distress from another, decide with pinpoint accuracy what treatment to prescribe, and confidently predict the outcome. Would that it were so!

Returning to autism, the early years of the diagnostic story were characterized by the steady accumulation of many case histories of children who broadly fitted Kanner's original criteria, but whose characteristic social difficulties could be accompanied by a whole array of different problems or patterns of unusual behaviour. Despite the use of the term 'autism' to describe the children's behaviour, in the 1940s and 50s, the early diagnostic manuals termed the condition 'childhood schizophrenia'. There was limited understanding of developmental psychiatric disorders at this stage, so clinicians fastened on existing adult categories, such as schizophrenia, and subsumed observations of 'matching' symptoms in children into the same category.

Attempts were made to improve the situation by producing some set of behavioural characteristics that might distinguish autism as a unique developmental problem. In the US, Bernard Rimland, a psychologist and autism researcher, developed the Rimland Diagnostic Form for Behaviour-Disturbed Children.[10] Limited eye contact or difficulty in maintaining relationships would serve as an example of impaired social interaction. In the UK, a diagnostic checklist also emerged in the early 1960s, thanks to the efforts of a British psychiatrist, Mildred Creak, who got together a panel of experts to see if they could devise an agreed-upon description of what types of behaviour were key to identifying what was then still being called 'schizophrenic syndrome of childhood'.[11]

Creak's Nine Points were published in 1961. Under the heading 'Schizophrenic syndrome in childhood', the group listed the standard Kanner-type signs concerning relationships with other people and sustained resistance to change, but also highlighted more specific behavioural problems, such as pathological preoccupation with particular objects, illogical anxiety, and strange movement patterns. Creak's group also noted poor or absent speech, and what was called 'islets of normal, near normal, or exceptional intellectual function'. By this time, the search for the psychoanalytical significance of these behaviours had virtually disappeared, and just the presence (or absence) of such unusual behaviours was used to arrive at a diagnosis.

Such checklists began to be widely used in clinical practice and research settings and brought some coherence to the study of autism. As a consequence, the concept of autism was officially recognized in 1980 in the DSM-3, the third edition of the American Psychiatric Association's *Diagnostic and Statistical Manual of Mental Disorders*.[12] It was included as 'infantile autism' under the heading 'Pervasive Developmental Disorders' (PDD), with the key feature remaining true to Kanner's focus on 'lack of social responsiveness'.

However, this official picture of autism began to change in the 1970s due to the efforts of the UK psychiatrist Lorna Wing and her colleague Judith Gould.[13] They were involved in a project to estimate the incidence of autism in the general population. Wing and Gould surveyed all the children in the London area of Camberwell with what we would now call 'learning difficulties.' In the first instance, their approach was to measure the incidence of physical behaviours associated with autism, such as hand-flapping or social aloofness, but also language abnormalities ranging from the nonverbal to the highly articulate, as well as the characteristic oddities of social behaviour.

But they did not pick only those children who had all the Kanner-type signs; they noted that there were children who did not show the characteristic extremes of unusual behaviour, or even the full range, but still presented as atypical. Some could be quite sociable but had unusual patterns of language use. For example, they might cheerfully and appropriately greet the researcher, but then lapse into very formalized language, such as saying, 'I am experiencing a sensation of dehydration and require fluid intake,' instead of 'I'm thirsty'. (Think of the Mr. Spock character in *Star Trek*, for example.) Wing referred to this presentation of autism as 'active but odd', individuals who could be socially engaging, but who were recognizably unusual or different.

I encountered this presentation in a boy in a special school in Essex I visited. He had been selected to greet an arriving dignitary due to open a new sports facility. He had been carefully coached as to the appropriate social distance, handshake, and 'respectful stance', and looked on course to make a successful ambassador for the centre. What was not taken into account, however, was that he was obsessed with television adverts, especially those for medical products, and knew hundreds of them by heart. When he was stressed, he would obsessively repeat them verbatim, sometimes for hours. It turned out that, despite the training, he was finding his ambassadorial role quite stressful. So the visiting celebrity was somewhat startled when, after the slight bow and handshake (and there may have been a bouquet involved), her escort earnestly enquired, 'Do you suffer from flatulence, bloating, or diarrhoea? Help is at hand'. (Luckily the visitor took this in her stride, thanking him warmly, and said she would certainly bear his advice in mind.)

Wing and colleagues felt that there was some kind of 'Kanner walled garden' into which some children could be admitted, but that there were many other children who were still impaired and in need of support, who weren't captured by the strict requirements of the Kanner label. Wing and Gould proposed a 'triad of impairments', consisting of three core areas of difficulty. At the heart of this newer incarnation of autism were still the problems with social interaction, such as difficulties in understanding social cues or forming relationships, together with the traditional repetitive behaviours, such as rocking or hand-flapping, or obsessive interests in unusual and narrow topics, as well as the resistance to change. But Wing and Gould added language and communication problems as another diagnostically significant aspect of autism. These could include delayed language development and/or extremely literal use of language. In one of the psychiatric hospitals I worked in, I had to remove the sign from my door that said 'Knock and Enter', as passing patients were constantly doing just that.

It was at this point that Asperger came into the story. Individual clinicians were aware of his work, but it had not yet been published in English. Lorna Wing was one of those clinicians: she found out as much as she could about his work and, in 1981, published an influential paper that aimed to introduce the concept of 'Asperger's syndrome' to the clinical world.[14] Asperger's observations about the highly intelligent but socially and behaviourally unusual children he had encountered in his clinic resonated well with Wing and Gould's findings. It also allowed a wider definition of what being autistic might mean. This more flexible category of autistic-like behaviour proved so popular that its enthusiastic application led to an explosion of diagnoses and talk of autism epidemics. Wing referred to it as opening Pandora's box.[15] The word 'autism' was indeed, Humpty Dumpty–like, coming to mean many different things.

Asperger's paper on 'autistic psychopathy' in childhood was subsequently translated into English by renowned psychologist and autism researcher Uta Frith in 1991, making his work widely accessible to autism researchers, clinicians, and advocates.[16] The notion of high-achieving 'little professors' resonated well with the *Rain Man* phenomenon emerging in the public understanding of what autism was, and it also added a positive spin to the generally stigmatized concept of mental illness. There was a considerable campaign to ensure that Asperger was granted his rightful place as a co-father of autism, and in DSM-4, published in 1994, this was achieved: Asperger's syndrome was added as a distinct diagnostic category.[17] Social difficulties were still core to the diagnosis, but there was an emphasis on intact language and cognitive skills. Indeed, the emerging picture was of unusually high-functioning individuals whose intense focus on high-level skills such as music or mathematics resulted in astonishing achievements. Interest developed in individual 'savants' such as Daniel Tammet and Stephen Wiltshire, as did something of a fashion for diagnoses of famous scientists and artists. A high-profile celebrity linked to Asperger's syndrome today is Greta Thunberg, proudly tweeting,

'I have Asperger's and that means I'm sometimes a bit different from the norm. And – given the right circumstances – being different is a superpower'.[18]

As well as heralding the addition of Asperger's syndrome, DSM-4 marked a significant reorganization for autism itself. It was no longer referred to as 'infantile autism' but rather grouped under the broader category of 'pervasive developmental disorders'. This category encompassed several specific disorders as well as 'Asperger's disorder', including 'autistic disorder', 'Rett's disorder', 'childhood disintegrative disorder', and the frustratingly vague 'pervasive developmental disorder not otherwise specified' (PDD-NOS). PDD-NOS appeared to be a home for developmental disorders you couldn't fit anywhere else, including 'atypical autism' – or in other words autism that didn't quite fulfil the clinical criteria for autism but was 'autism-like'. The autism community sometimes referred to this diagnosis as 'Paediatrician Didn't Decide'.

Autistic disorder involved difficulties in three increasingly familiar patterns of behaviour: in social interaction, in language and communication, and in restricted or repetitive patterns of behaviour. In an impressive array of what looked like diagnostic specificity, sixteen additional items were listed under the three impairment headings – such as 'lack of awareness of the existence or feelings of others', 'lack of interest in stories about imaginary events', and 'persistent preoccupation with parts of objects'. But the feeling that one might at last be heading towards a distinctive picture of autism starts to unravel when you learn that only eight out of these sixteen criteria had to be present, of which two (but only two) must come from each of the major categories. It is not hard to see that you could quite quickly gather a collection of children, all of whom fulfilled the criteria for having an autistic disorder but had quite different behavioural profiles. No wonder the autistic community has a famous saying: 'If you've met one person with autism, you've met one person with autism'![19]

Having worked through the DSM-4 checklist, scanning an enormously long list of signs of a given disorder, you might find – just when you felt you were on the home stretch towards a final diagnosis – a rider asking you to check that 'criteria are not met for another pervasive developmental disorder or schizophrenia'.

It is perhaps the story of a totally new member of this diagnostic family that reveals how far we still were, even with the attempted clarifications in DSM-4, from providing a definitive answer to the question of what autism actually is. This was Rett syndrome – characterized by normal development for the first six months of life at which time nearly all language and motor skills were lost, with clear signs of severe intellectual disability and lack of social skills. The behavioural symptoms of Rett were sufficiently similar to those of autism that it was decided that it fitted alongside autistic disorder in the category of pervasive developmental disorders. This decision was clarified by Fred Volkmar, a Yale professor of child psychiatry, paediatrics, and psychology, one of the key players in the development of DSM-4 (and, indeed, DSM-5), in terms that perhaps reveal the sometimes fuzzy thinking behind the diagnostic checklists in such manuals. 'Rett's disorder was included because it *appeared* to be a very interesting condition that *might* have a specific neurobiological basis and the PDDs (Pervasive Developmental Disorders) *seemed* the best place for it' (italics are my emphases), wrote Volkmar.[20] In a further touch of smoke and mirrors, Rett syndrome disappeared in the next edition of DSM as its genetic bases had been identified. Since it had a biomarker, it didn't count as a psychiatric issue any more.

The DSM-4's heroic attempt to neatly slot different manifestations into subcategories revealed the wide variety of different behavioural patterns that characterized those who might (or might not) be called autistic. This did not play out well with clinicians, who tried to follow the complicated choice points to a hopefully useful diagnosis. I once went birdwatching with a friend who regaled me with the number of different shades of brown that could be used to describe the birds flitting past the hide window. I managed 'light brown', 'dark brown', and 'reddish brown', but lost the plot when we got to 'taupe', 'sepia', 'mottled brown', and 'streaked brown'. I could manage 'big', 'small', 'brown', and 'black', but I never got the hang of 'what kind of brown'. My struggles with trying to understand just what distinguished one brown from another seemed to exactly capture the difficulties the well-meaning subcategorization of autism was causing. Can the term 'autism' really be applied to so many different things?

THE ROAD TO DSM-5

By the beginning of this century, it had become clear that autism (however specified) was a highly heritable condition. By looking at the increased likelihood of siblings of autistic children also being autistic, by studying twins with autism, by studying the incidence of autism-like characteristics in the wider family, it became clear to researchers that a high proportion of autism's characteristics could be attributed to genetic influences. This new understanding made it increasingly important for the autism world to come to some kind of agreement as to what autism actually was. Geneticists were keen to identify 'autism genes'; neuroscientists like me were keen to 'profile' the autistic brain; psychologists were devising experimental paradigms so they could explore the core manifestations of autism. Researchers of all stripes were calling for a reliable and consistent picture of what it was they were studying – they needed to be certain they were recruiting subjects from a clearly defined population. But exactly what was the difference between typical and atypical autism? Could a UK researcher be sure that her colleagues in the US were studying children with the same pattern of problems? And was Asperger's really different from so-called high-functioning autism?

There was still evidence that decisions about who was or was not autistic varied quite dramatically in different locations, quite often linked to what help might become available if a child was given a clinical diagnosis. There is a comment from psychiatrist Judy Rapoport that is often quoted: 'I'll call a kid a zebra if it will get him the educational services I think he needs'.[21] In the United States, insurance plans were now legally required to cover autism therapies, so getting a diagnosis (or not) had financial implications. In addition, the notion of a broad autism phenotype was emerging, suggesting that individuals might have a 'touch of autism', or could display autistic-like traits, such as restricted interests or social awkwardness, that didn't quite fit into the existing classification system. In short, the term 'autism' was being bandied about even more freely.

The Neurodevelopmental Disorders Workgroup convened to discuss what needed to be done to resolve such matters in the next issue of DSM. Was it time to move away from the long-held belief in autism as a specific distinct category and think about it more as a dimension or 'spectrum', as Lorna Wing had long wanted it described? Did the range of symptoms reported still fit comfortably into a triad structure, requiring several ticks in three separate boxes to reach a diagnosis? And what about complaints that one of the most characteristic aspects of autistic behaviour, those of enhanced or reduced sensory sensitivities, were not part of the definition? Statisticians, researchers, and clinicians pored over the many different measures that existed to see if they could come up with a set of criteria that would better answer the 'what is autism?' question. And so, in 2013, DSM-5 arrived.

On the surface, streamlining seemed to triumph in DSM-5. Gone were the five different categories (including Asperger's syndrome), and a single umbrella term, called 'autism spectrum disorder', emerged. Autism was no longer associated with three types of difficulties – it was now two. Atypical social behaviour in all its forms was one of the major headings, with three subcategories that had to be evident for a diagnosis. These included problems such as difficulties in maintaining relationships and failure to follow implicit conversational rules. Autism assessments should now be focussed on positioning individuals along a dimension rather than slotting them into separate categories. The phrase 'on the spectrum' now entered public discourse when referring to someone who had been diagnosed as autistic or who showed autistic tendencies.

DSM-5 also made an explicit reference to the possibility of autism emerging later in someone's developmental history. Although the earlier, more rigid requirement that the problems had to emerge in the first three years of life had been dropped in the 1980s, as well as the term 'infantile autism', the picture had remained of autism as a problem of early development. Now we were told that the diagnostic characteristics 'may not become fully manifest until social demands exceed limited capacities'. It was now possible for someone not to be diagnosed as autistic until they were an adult. This was quite a marked shift in the picture of autism, which, to date, had been a childhood disorder.

The other heading in this newer binary approach to autism was that of 'restricted, repetitive patterns of behaviour, interests or activities' (abbreviated to RRBIs).[22] A wide range of problems were grouped under this heading, including the stereotypical hand-flapping or rocking, the insistence on sameness, and the abnormally intense focus on unusual objects. You may find these two behavioural categories uncannily reminiscent of Kanner's original headings, nearly seventy years earlier.

Sensory problems at last made an appearance, under RRBIs. The rationale was that sometimes children's stereotyped movements such as rocking or hand-flapping can be set off by bright lights or loud sounds. Or the obsessive sniffing or touching of objects shown by some autistic children could count as a manifestation of repetitive behaviours. Some have claimed that this nod to sensory problems appears to have been shoehorned in, but its inclusion has been welcomed by most (especially as this symptom 'footnote' may be more characteristic of females than males on the spectrum).

The new DSM also includes a severity rating for each of the various problem areas, ranging from level 3, 'requiring very substantial support', through level 2, 'requiring substantial support', to level 1, 'requiring support'. But here things get a little blurry again – what exactly differs between substantial and very substantial? As a researcher interested in sensory difficulties in autism, I thought it might be useful to further explore the different grades that this new system could allocate. Learning that 'substantial support' was associated with difficulties appearing 'frequently enough to be obvious to the casual observer' didn't seem to offer me the kind of specifics that might be useful in selecting participants for my studies or working out how best to analyze their data.

We might take a sideways step at this point and consider why understanding the hits and misses en route to a clear-cut description of autism is important. If the right label can be clearly linked to the best advice about recognition and prognosis, and to the best kind of treatments and interventions, it is obviously important for clinicians. If the right label can help parents and carers understand the bewildering array of problems with which their autistic child is presenting them, then the necessity is equally obvious. If the label can allow a researcher to neatly cluster their participants into autistic or non-autistic groups, then the geneticists can pursue their explorations; neuroscientists can start profiling autistic brains; and endocrinologists and biochemists can examine brain-body-behaviour links. But it turns out that, in addition, with respect to autism in particular, a precise label can confer a welcome sense of identity to autistic individuals themselves.

The value of this sense of identity is well characterized by tracking the appearance, the moment in the spotlight, and the subsequent disappearance of Asperger's syndrome as a diagnosis.

WHATEVER HAPPENED TO ASPERGER'S SYNDROME?

In 2013, the term 'Asperger's syndrome' was dropped from the fifth edition of the DSM. The condition was to be subsumed under the new heading 'autism spectrum disorder'. A year or so earlier, I was attending a workshop on integrating individuals with mental health problems into the workplace, which included vigorous advocacy for the recognition and support of individuals with Asperger's syndrome. Having been peripherally involved in the consultations leading up to the DSM-5 changes, I mentioned (helpfully, I thought) the upcoming disappearance of that particular label, flagging the need to be aware that a different term was going to emerge. This was apparently news to most of the audience.

The reaction was a bit like those twentieth-century UK cartoons by H. M. Bateman depicting extremes of outrage, shock, and consternation caused by some kind of social faux pas: 'The Man Who . . . Passed the Port the Wrong Way'/'Asked for a Second Helping at a Company Dinner'/'Failed to Stand Up for the National Anthem'. (Non-UK readers might like to check out the website www.hmbateman.com/gallery/the-man-who-.htm to get a feel for this quintessentially British sense of humour. Or ponder how social gaffes are characterized in their own cultures.) It was as though I had indicated that preparations were in hand to arrange the worldwide disappearance of all individuals who had been diagnosed with Asperger's syndrome (or, indeed, that I was personally responsible for such preparations). The Q and A session was monopolized by indignant comments:

> 'I fought for years to get my son diagnosed as Asperger's and now you're telling me it doesn't exist.'

> 'Being told I had Asperger's Syndrome meant my life suddenly made sense and now you're going to take that away from me.'

> 'If I'm not an Aspie then what am I?'

A colleague on the same panel muttered that it might be better if I didn't join the audience in the coffee break, and the organizers swiftly announced that we had overrun on time and there would be no more Q and As.

Once the DSM-5 changes became official, my own experience was mirrored in many public fora, with widespread outcries along the lines of 'DSM-5 is taking away our identity' and vigorous opposition from online communities such as Wrong Planet.[23] There was some concern that the DSM-5 change could cause a tightening of the diagnostic net and subsequent loss of benefits. But most concern seemed to be with losing a label about which some kind of public awareness had been established, bringing an understanding of, or explanation for, unusual or possibly isolating patterns of behaviour.

The Asperger's story rumbles on. Rather oddly, although Asperger's syndrome as a diagnostic term disappeared in 2013 with the new DSM edition, it remained in the *International Statistical Classification of Diseases* manual until 2021.[24] So there was a little window of opportunity where you could still be an 'Aspie' although officially it was no longer a 'thing'. We mentioned earlier that Greta Thunberg had referred to her Asperger's as her superpower. Behavioural scientists have tracked the impact of the Thunberg–Asperger's link on public interest in autism.[25] They monitored internet searches for Asperger's syndrome during the time she spoke at the UN Climate Action Summit in September 2019 and found that online searches had climbed to 1,300,997, an increase of 254.07 per cent from the level predicted by previous search activity. This was taken as a positive sign, that a particular diagnostic label attached to a high-profile individual could increase interest in, and understanding of, just what that label meant.

What began as a clinical term, or a diagnostic label, had become an issue of identity. Having a diagnosis such as Asperger's was really important to its recipient, not necessarily with respect to insurance coverage or protected characteristics, but for the fact that it signalled membership in a clearly defined 'tribe', in this case one that proudly called itself Aspies. It was a label that had a (mainly) positive place in public consciousness, and awareness of Asperger's and what it meant could bring with it allowances for characteristic oddities that may previously have led to social rejection or isolation.

Knowing what such labels mean, then, is about more than the accurate slotting of an individual into the 'right' mental health category; it is about giving someone a personal and social identity, about what such labels mean to the person to whom they are now attached. As we will see in the next chapter, the issue of losing the term 'Asperger's' from the autism catalogue was more than just a clinical decision, but it does illustrate the fact that labels can matter beyond their presence in a diagnostic manual. And it also means that those who are denied the label, for whatever reason, are also denied a chance to find a 'tribe' to which they might belong.

This brings us to the issue of how you actually 'earn' the autism label – what specific measures are used to decide that a child (or an adult) presenting with a set of behavioural problems is 'on the spectrum'. As yet there is no so-called biomarker, a defining physical feature that could reliably and objectively confirm an autism diagnosis. So it is necessary to find a way of devising measures that can reliably capture the essence of autistic behaviours, including the extent to which they are different from some kind of agreed-upon norm. Over time, and alongside the ever-changing picture of autism, elaborate testing systems have been devised. If you have taken your child for an autism assessment, or if you yourself have been referred to have one, you will have encountered such tests.

DIAGNOSING AUTISM: WHAT GETS MEASURED?

Early accounts of what we now call autism comprised case by case descriptions of individual children, published by clinicians such as Kanner. Other clinicians would then consult these in order to find comparisons with their own patients. Kanner and Asperger had provided immensely detailed observations, not only of the immediate problems of the children they were studying, but also comments on their birth experiences and early years' development, and descriptions of childhood illnesses. They also included quite judgemental details on the children's parents and grandparents and their family histories. Kanner, for example, noted that the father of Alfred 'does not get along well with people, . . . spends his spare time reading, gardening and fishing', whereas his mother 'is a "clinical psychologist", very obsessive and excitable'.[26]

But such painstaking and elaborate history taking did not reveal the kind of consistent patterns of problems that all the children had in common, which might then have allowed clinicians to identify a reliable grouping or diagnostic category into which the children might fit. Rimland's and Creak's checklists were the beginning of this approach, but their definitions were still rather vague. How, for example, might you measure 'apparent unawareness of his own identity', from the Creak checklist?

Once autism was recognized as a specific disorder in DSM-3, it became clear that some kind of standardized protocols were required to give a better view of what any autistic child was really like. An agreed-upon diagnostic test was needed, with a set of questions to ask or activities to observe. Ideally, the measure would be the same wherever someone was being assessed, and could yield a numerical score that would tell the same story. Such tests began to emerge in the late 1980s. Their aim was challenging – to discriminate autism from any other kind of disabilities. There were already some rating scales around, but it was felt by clinicians and educators that they didn't discriminate enough from other developmental disorders.

The need for more valid and reliable instruments led to the emergence of the so-called 'gold standard' tests: the Autism Diagnostic Observation Schedule (ADOS) and the Autism Diagnostic Interview (ADI).[27] These are the most widely recognized tests for autism in use today, developed mainly for use with children but adaptable for adults. Hand in hand with the ongoing attempts to find a definition of autism, these tests were the product of exhaustive trialling of ways to measure the key features of autistic behaviour. What behavioural atypicalities seemed to be most characteristic of those children who had been identified as autistic? What aspects of their developmental history seemed to be most predictive of who did or didn't get an autism diagnosis?

The ADOS (and its subsequent revisions) is activity based and made up of a set of standardized scenarios to monitor how an individual communicates and interacts with other people. With a young child, this may involve watching how they play and if they show signs of imagination (are they happy pretending a wooden brick is a truck, for example?). Older children may be asked about experiences at school or friendships. They are also analyzed for any signs of unusual movement patterns or obsessive focus on favourite topics. It can take a long time to go through all the different tasks, carefully following the standardized protocols, which is part of the explanation for the extraordinarily long waiting lists for a formal autism diagnosis. There are four different modules – total scores range from fifteen to sixty, with a cut-off score of thirty and above to indicate autism.

The ADI is an interview schedule involving the parents or carers of potentially autistic individuals being asked to describe the subjects' differences or difficulties. It involves ninety-three (ninety-three!) different questions about communication and language skills, social interaction, and evidence of repetitive or obsessive behaviours, and can take over two hours to administer. A score is generated for social behaviour, language development, and restricted range of interests or stereotyped behaviours. For example, there are fifteen different questions about social behaviour – you need to score at least ten for this to count towards an autism assessment.

ADOS and ADI tests have become near compulsory if you are trying to create an education support plan for a child on the spectrum, or bid to a funding body for research in the autism field, or identify special provisions for an employee, or access some kind of therapeutic support. They are widely praised for high levels of reliability and validity.

However, we should definitely note the framing of the scoring criteria. For example, 'social communication should be below *that expected* for general developmental level'; 'fixated interests are *abnormal* in intensity or focus (e.g., strong attachment to or preoccupation with *unusual* objects' (italics are my emphasis). Bearing in mind that answers are based on self-reports from parents or carers or teachers, if not autistic individuals themselves, we might like to ask what determines whether something is 'below expected', 'abnormal', or 'unusual'? No specific quantitative norms are provided.

Interview schedules such as the ADI for children may be dependent on what parents/caregivers can remember of their child's early years and their interpretation of what the questions they are being asked actually mean. If someone asks a parent, 'Does your child find it easy to make friends?', does this mean compared to her/his siblings, to your own experience or expectations? Should they consider what her/his teachers have been telling them, or recall comments from well-meaning/judgemental people in the supermarket? If the person being assessed is an adult, then their answers may be based on even older memories, perhaps associated with troubling events in their early years, or the answers may be biased by the hope that the tests might give them the answers they are looking for. To further complicate matters, we know that autism is highly heritable and can often run undetected in families for years, especially in older generations. This may well be reflected in the very family histories that those being diagnosed are asked to explore. So if you are the parent seeking diagnosis for an autistic child, or an adult seeking diagnosis for yourself, how much more different might your sense of 'normal' childhood behaviour be compared to that of a neurotypical person?

An enormous amount of clinical experience and expertise has gone into the development of such tests and their use has provided some valuable consistency to ongoing attempts to find an accurate answer to the question of 'What is autism?' But, as we shall see, there is still a considerable way to go, particularly with regard to how reliably these tests identify the experience of women and girls.

WHAT DOES AUTISM LOOK LIKE? THE AUTISM PHENOTYPE

We have looked at the history of autism, tracked its entrance into psychiatry's weighty diagnostic tomes, and followed the emergence of elaborate measuring instruments. But has this told us what it might be like to meet an individual 'on the spectrum'? Obviously parents and carers will have their own tales to tell about what autism looks like. Professional manuals such as DSM-5 describe autism as 'persistent difficulties with social communication and social interaction, restricted and repetitive patterns of behaviours, activities or interests to the extent that these limit and impair everyday functioning'. But what does that mean? If you were a teacher anticipating the arrival of an autistic child in your class, or an employer about to interview someone who had 'declared' their autism, or someone about to meet an autistic member of a friend's family, what might you expect that person to be like? Perhaps this might be a better window onto the answer to the 'what is autism?' question.

You might already know something about the difficulties with social engagement that people with autism experience, the likelihood that they will come across as aloof or standoffish. This behaviour is often stereotypically characterized as 'lack of eye contact' (still found on some UK National Health Service [NHS] websites today as a sign of autism). Measures of social responsiveness offer between sixty-five and one hundred ways of assessing odd social behaviours, including whether or not an individual will join group activities without being told to do so, or knows when they are invading someone's personal space.[28]

You might also expect some unusual actions such as rocking or hand-flapping; various surveys on public perception of autism commonly identify these as most commonly associated with autism. Similarly, obsessive rituals (lining up toys in colour order, or books in height order) and insistence on specific routines might figure. You might look out for highly focussed interests – train spotting still heads lists of allegedly characteristic autistic behaviour – or fascination with obscure facts about car engines.

But a common expectation about this autistic individual that you are about to encounter is that they will be male. In order to fully understand autism, we need to understand how and why this expectation came about, and how much it has shaped (or even distorted) the whole autism story.

CHAPTER 2

AUTISM'S MALE SPOTLIGHT PROBLEM

IN NEARLY EVERY AUTISM-RELATED CLINICAL MANUAL, research paper, website, and mainstream media opinion piece there will an assertion that autism is four times (and it is almost always four times) more common in boys than girls. This observed preponderance of males in autistic populations has become an additional defining characteristic of the condition. The notion that 'autism is a boy thing' has served as a long-standing framework, or spotlight, in all spheres of autism-related issues, from recognition and diagnosis through to public awareness and stereotypical media presentation, to theoretical models as well as cutting-edge research agendas. The consequences for our early understanding of autism fit well with Noam Chomsky's pithy observation about the problem of bias in science:

> Science is a bit like the joke about the drunk who is looking under a lamppost for the key he has lost on the other side of the street, because that is where the light is.[1]

When the English-speaking world was first made aware of what we now call autism, clinicians appeared to pay no particular attention to whether the cases they were reporting were male or female. Kanner's original cohort of eleven children included three girls – Barbara, Elaine, and Virginia. He certainly didn't comment on this eight–three split, although later researchers have. With the benefit of hindsight, this very early 8:3 ratio has sometimes been taken by epidemiologists, clinicians, and researchers as an early example of sex differences in the occurrence of autism. Once Asperger's work became available to the English-speaking world in the 1980s, his almost exclusive focus on boys was noted by several key players in the developing understanding of autism, including Lorna Wing, as it resonated well with emerging epidemiological commentaries about the male:female ratio in autism. Indeed, Asperger explicitly drew attention to the 'maleness' of autism, describing some of the subjects' odd behaviours and skills as characteristic of 'extreme male intelligence'. But we now know there could have been a darker reason for the absence of girls in Asperger's cohort.

ASPERGER'S MISSING GIRLS

Hans Asperger claimed that he had 'never met a girl with the fully fledged picture of autism'.[2] This statement, together with the fact that the four case histories Asperger presented in his first published study of 'autistic psychopathy' were all boys, seems to be the origin of the impression that autism is a condition found mainly, if not exclusively, in males. But it turns out that Asperger's claim was not wholly truthful. He did see girls, one of whom he actually referred to as 'severely autistic, very inaccessible from the outside'.[3] Recently excavated case notes revealed that several of the girls he saw showed startlingly similar behavioural profiles to the boys he wrote about, particularly the four boys he presented in his 1944 thesis – the cornerstone of what came to be called 'Asperger's syndrome'.[4]

Asperger's assessment of these girls was in the context of his role as director of the Curative Education Clinic in Vienna during the Third Reich. Shockingly, there is strong evidence that this clinic was a core part of the regime's child 'euthanasia' programme. Children's 'educability' was assessed here by clinicians, including Asperger. Any deemed irremediable could be sent to 'special hospitals', where they were made available to brutal and often fatal ongoing research experiments, and where the children were frequently murdered. One of the worst such facilities was Am Spiegelgrund, in Vienna. At least 789 children were murdered there during the Third Reich. There is evidence that dozens of them had been referred there by Asperger himself. This was unearthed by Edith Sheffer, a US historian specializing in German history, who found Asperger's district Nazi Party file and painstakingly tracked his story through hospital records and historical archives.[5] Sheffer was following up on the work of an Austrian historian, Herwig Czech, who had 'outed' Asperger's active involvement with National Socialism and its policies of eugenicist mass murder, at a symposium on Asperger's life and legacy.[6]

Up until 2010, there had been a long-standing impression, encouraged by Asperger himself, that he had acted as something of a psychiatric Schindler, emphasizing the special gifts of his 'little professors', thus heroically (and at some personal risk) keeping them out of the clutches of the 'special' children's wards. But it appears he was equally capable of marking children down as suitable only for elimination. For example, in one signed letter to the medical authorities, he notes that a three-year-old girl must be an 'unbearable burden' to her family and recommends 'permanent placement' at Am Spiegelgrund. Which is where she was sent and killed only two months later.

The four boys that Asperger wrote about were variously supported with special education programmes and survived the war. His 'imprimatur' could well have served as a protective mechanism of some kind. There is no evidence that he ever offered the same protection to any girls.

Were there no girls worth saving? No female 'little professors'? Edith Sheffer points out the startling similarities to Asperger's four boys in the behavioural profiles of two girls in particular, Elfriede and Margarete, also assessed by Asperger.[7] Reference was made to the boys' inability to form genuine human relationships. He noted an equivalent inability of Elfriede and Margarete to participate in the community of children and to misread social cues. Asperger appeared to interpret the same idiosyncrasies in the children differently. If you recall, Asperger commented on the 'advanced' use of language by Harro, one of the four boys in his 1944 paper. Harro's strange sentences and odd neologisms were referred to as 'autistic introspections', a sign of superior intelligence, while Margarete's lengthy monologues were dismissed as 'mannered and awkward'. Asperger made great efforts to get some kind of measure of the boys' intelligence; there is no record of any such assessment for the girls.

It may well be that the different societal standards for boys and girls contributed to the omission:

> In the heavily gendered expectations of boys' and girls' behaviour in the Third Reich, what mattered was girls' competence in private life, in domestic duties and personal relationships – and boys' competence in public life, in discipline, achievement, and peer integration.[8]

Fritz, Harro, Ernst, and Hellmuth were deemed worthy of intense therapeutic support and education, whereas both Elfriede and Margarete were deemed ineducable, of no social worth, unlikely to ever successfully perform 'domestic duties' or form 'personal relationships'. So they were sent off to Am Spiegelgrund. The 'ineducable' Elfriede wrote letters to both her mother and her uncle telling them that she felt these might be the last letters she would send. We know this because both letters are still in her file, presumably because Asperger's clinic never sent them on before she was dispatched to Spiegelgrund. According, again, to Edith Sheffer, 'Elfriede was deeply fearful about where [Asperger's] ward might send her'.

There is no record of either girl dying at the facility. We lose sight of Elfriede, but it emerges that Margarete survived her first visit, which was then followed by a round of different institutionalizations, including one where she was forcibly sterilized, then back on the assessment roundabout, including Asperger's clinic and Spiegelgrund again, at which point she was assessed as 'tentatively educable'. After that, there is no record.

'It is fascinating to note that the autistic children we have seen are almost exclusively boys'.[9] This statement by Asperger has left a legacy in the history of autism. It is important that those who still make reference to it – and the so-called father of autism's legacy – are aware of the context.[10]

There is another intriguing thread in the 'autism is a boy thing' story that should give us pause for thought in any debate about the origins of this belief. It turns out there was another earlier entry in the autism story than that provided by Kanner or Asperger. It has emerged that neither of these so-called 'father(s) of autism' were the first to record observations about the condition. The earliest reports of autism were by a female Soviet child psychiatrist.

THE 'MOTHER OF AUTISM'

In 1926 and 1927, about twenty years before either Kanner's or Asperger's paper appeared, Grunya Efimovna Sukhareva, a female Soviet child psychiatrist, published four highly detailed articles about children – six boys and five girls – whom she had encountered in her work in psychiatric clinics in present-day Ukraine.[11] She initially referred to 'schizoid psychopathy' but later renamed the condition as 'autistic psychopathy'.

Sukhareva offers wonderfully detailed, painstaking descriptions of each of her patients, having observed them over several years in the hospital-schools she had helped to set up, specifically to offer help and training to struggling children. Her meticulous clinical notes include family histories and physical characteristics, but, most particularly, the behaviour of these children. There is little evidence of intellectual disability in any of the cases she grouped together – in fact, she often seemed to be at pains to draw attention to their musical or artistic skills – but their behaviour had become sufficiently unmanageable that they had been admitted to a clinic.

All of her patients had unusual patterns of high and low levels of ability, what Sukhareva called 'a mixture of finesse and silliness'. One boy, with an apparently limited and monotonous style of speaking, and a tendency to ask 'absurd' questions, when asked if he liked the book he was reading, replied, 'I think I liked the book, but I'm not really sure; the principle of reading is such that you are absorbed'. A 'failure to connect' with their classmates appeared to be a universal feature in all of these children, which Sukhareva, significantly, referred to as the result of an 'autistic and withdrawn attitude'.

Sukhareva drew attention to the differences between the boys and the girls she was writing about, publishing separate papers on them and then summarizing the 'specific particularities' that distinguished them. The main difference was that disordered emotional or affective behaviour was always at the forefront of the female picture, with 'bizarre and contradictory' variabilities of mood. One girl, described as 'sensitive, tender and kind', would suddenly show inexplicable and unpredictable outbursts of rudeness and defiance. Sukhareva describes another girl as able to 'vividly and compassionately understand others'. This presentation in girls was compared to patterns of thinking more characteristic of boys, with their eccentric trains of thought, and obsessive fascination with specific processes such as mathematical calculations or specific historical events. The boys' emotional behaviour was more likely to be characterized by apathy or indifference, or active avoidance of their classmates. She concludes, 'The general picture of schizoid psychopathies is paler in girls than in boys, and the schizoid peculiarities appear less marked. Also the percentage of schizoid psychopathies seem to be lower in girls'.

With these observations, predating Kanner and Asperger by a couple of decades, Grunya Efimovna Sukhareva provided a meticulous picture of behaviour in both girls and boys, who could be grouped together by one defining characteristic, their 'autistic' and withdrawn attitude. But, even more importantly to the theme of this book, Sukhareva not only acknowledged the presence of girls, but also catalogued differences between them and the boys she observed. But then she disappeared from the autism story altogether until the end of the last century.

During the nearly fifty years after Kanner drew attention to autistic behaviour in children, Sukhareva appeared nowhere in any subsequent discussions or diagnostic developments. In 1996, Sula Wolff, a child psychiatrist, herself working with recognizably autistic children whom she described as 'loners', translated part of Sukhareva's early work into English, in a paper entitled, 'The first account of the syndrome Asperger described?'[12] But Wolff, inexplicably, only translated the work on boys. Perhaps her decision was linked to the current enthusiasm for Asperger and his insistence on the 'boy' picture of autism.

It was not as if her observations of autistic children were old-fashioned or outdated or failed to match up with those that appeared afterwards. In their 2015 paper decrying the lack of recognition of Sukhareva in the history of autism, Swedish psychiatric researchers Irina Manouilenko and Susanne Bejerot pointed out the astonishing similarities between Sukhareva's descriptions of her child patients and DSM-5's criteria for the diagnosis of ASD.[13] For example, her description of her children's 'autistic attitude: tendency towards solitude and avoidance of other people from early childhood onwards; avoids company with other children' maps presciently onto DSM-5's 'persistent deficits in social communication and social interaction across multiple contexts; . . . deficits in developing, maintaining and understanding relationships'. Sukhareva was way ahead of her time.

So why hasn't Sukhareva been christened the 'mother of autism' and why did we overlook her prescient observations about females? Perhaps because she was not as well known outside of her country, although it is hard to believe her high profile within the Soviet Union did not attract some attention elsewhere. She had a lengthy career as a psychiatrist, practising from 1917 to 1969, established many hospital-school clinics, headed up several different psychiatry departments, and was the recipient of numerous awards in recognition of her work, including the Order of Lenin, the Order of the Badge of Honour, and the title Honoured Scientist of the RSFSR (Russian Soviet Federative Socialist Republic).[14]

It could be that working in the Soviet Union and publishing mainly in Russian was a barrier, making her work less accessible – linguistically and politically – in Western countries, especially the US. However, Sukhareva did also publish her work on both boys and girls in German (the native language of both Leo Kanner and Hans Asperger). In fact, Kanner himself cited her later work and there is evidence that she corresponded with him. However, he remained resolutely silent on the evidence that she had predated his own work on autism by some twenty years. It has been suggested that Hans Asperger in particular could well have come across her papers; indeed, he referred to other papers published in the same German-language journals that she published in.

After Sula Wolff informed the scientific community about Sukhareva's work on autistic boys, we had to wait until 2019 for the Soviet psychiatrist's observations about autistic girls to be published, as part of a thesis on her place in the history of autism research. Charlotte Simmonds, the author of the paper, thoughtfully added Sukhareva as her co-author.[15] This acknowledgement was not extended to others who previously drew on her research! Coincidentally, Kevin Rebecchi, a French psychology professor, also produced an independently published book containing English translations of the German versions of Sukhareva's papers on autistic children. Its cover excitedly describes it as 'A text that is still relevant almost 100 years after it was written!'[16]

Eventually (but not until 2023), researchers David Sher and Jenny Gibson drew the Sukhareva threads together in their survey of her work, not just on autism but also on her contribution to psychiatry as a whole.[17] In a paper enthusiastically entitled 'Pioneering, Prodigious and Perspicacious: Grunya Efimovna Sukhareva's Life and Contribution to Conceptualising Autism and Schizophrenia', they nominated her 1920s papers as describing the first clinical account of autistic children and note (at last!) that she was ahead of her time in her focus on females, acknowledging the importance of her observations about the differing manifestations of autism in girls.

It took almost exactly one hundred years before we got to hear about the seminal work of a female psychiatrist writing about autistic females. Since then, clinicians and psychiatric historians have commented on the 'amazing precision and modernity' of Sukhareva's work, claiming that she had actually beaten Kanner to the punch (and possibly been plagiarized by Asperger). They have likewise demanded her rightful place in the autism story be recognized.

We don't know why Sukhareva was written out of autism's history. Perhaps the two most powerful male figures were just in the right place at the right time. Kanner was certainly ambitious with respect to making a reputation in psychiatry and not shy of claiming first place in the 'discovery' of autism. There is less evidence that Asperger was after this sort of acclaim, but he appears to have had a powerful set of advocates (perhaps as much anti-Kanner as pro-Asperger) who wanted to make sure Kanner didn't get all the glory. The jury is still out on whether either or both of them deliberately chose to ignore Sukhareva's work or were genuinely unaware of it. But neither of them ever offered any kind of retrospective acknowledgement of what she had had to say, some twenty years before their 'breakthrough' publications.

Even those stoutly advocating for Sukhareva's belated recognition are sometimes guilty of overlooking her contributions to the study of autism in females. Ironically, in the introduction to her paper on girls, she noted, 'The problem of the influence of sex differences on the symptomatology and course of various clinical forms deserves much more attention than it usually receives'. Indeed!

AUTISM IS A BOY THING: FAIR COMMENT?

Although some insights into origins of the notion of autism as being primarily a male problem may be found lurking in the shadows of autism history, maleness did not become the core defining characteristic until sometime after its entry into clinical diagnoses. The 1940s and 1950s saw the emergence of autism advocacy movements, commonly initiated by parents of autistic children who were often fighting against compulsory institutionalization or for the right of their children to have access to education. These children, on whose behalf families were taking up the cudgels, were just as likely to be daughters as sons. For example, Clara Claiborne Park, the American activist and author, wrote her 1967 bestseller *The Siege*, about her experiences with her daughter Jessy. The psychiatrist and researcher Lorna Wing, who, as we know, was one of the key players in the development of our modern-day understanding of autism, was also the mother of a severely autistic daughter, Susie. The anthropologist Roy Richard Grinker, who used his academic expertise to dispel the myths associated with the worldwide increase in diagnoses of autism, got involved in the debate partly in response to the diagnosis of his daughter, Isabel, in 1994. One of today's leading autism neuroscience researchers, Kevin Pelphrey, from Yale University's NIH Autism Center for Excellence, has written of how the autism diagnosis of his daughter, Frances, at age three, determined the subsequent focus of his research. In all of these stories, no one seems to have been taking any notice of whether they were talking about sons or daughters, brothers or sisters.[18]

But the numbers were starting to tell a story. Kanner did not initially draw attention to any male bias, but by 1955, when reporting on the accumulating cases of 'his' syndrome, he did refer to a consistent preponderance of boys over girls, in a ratio of four to one.[19] He did not appear to attach any particular significance to this, although, in the concluding part of his report, he did rather oddly comment that research had failed to find any physical abnormalities to explain autism 'unless one considers relevant the consistent preponderance of boys over girls in a ratio of 4 to 1'. He doesn't clarify what kind of abnormalities might be associated with being a boy or a girl!

Was this just an anecdotal impression, then, or was it borne out by epidemiological evidence? Once some kind of agreed-upon checklist of what autism might look like had been arrived at, it became possible to do a headcount of all the cases of autism that had been identified, from which epidemiologists might then be able to extract some kind of pattern as to any defining characteristics of such populations.

The first attempt at a proper epidemiological survey took place in the UK, published in 1966.[20] You might find it surprising that the original estimate of autism's prevalence was based on a heroic headcount within the entire population of eight- to ten-year-olds in the county of Middlesex in the UK. Victor Lotter, a psychologist based at the Institute of Psychiatry in London, contacted every school and mental hospital in Middlesex with a questionnaire about behavioural peculiarities shown by the children in their care. His list was derived from a combination of Kanner's writing and Creak's Nine Points. He calmly points out in his paper that this involved contacts for 76,388 children, of whom he managed to get 75,930 reports (remember, this was before the days of email and online surveys).

Lotter and his research assistant (his wife, Ann) then identified 135 children who fulfilled the Kanner and Creak criteria, who were then visited and issued a range of developmental tests. With seventy-four eliminated as not fitting all of the criteria, the Lotters finally had a list of sixty-one possibles. Children then received scores on each of the items on the Lotters' behavioural checklist – either 0 (absent), 1 (present but not markedly), or 2 (markedly present). We should remember that, at this stage, these decisions were being made by just two researchers, the husband and wife team. This is not to suggest any data fixing or deliberate bias took place, but it certainly wasn't a double- or even single-blind clinical trial. And finally, ranking the sixty-one sets of scores from high to low, they then decided to divide the dataset in half (with no rationale given). The 'top' thirty-two children were deemed 'autistic', and the remaining children were labeled 'non-autistic' (you may wonder what the difference between cases 32 and 33 might have been – it is not given in the paper). And so the Lotters came up with a figure of 4.1 per 10,000 (or 0.04 per cent) as the first estimate of the prevalence of autism (with no discussion as to the representativeness of Middlesex or the accuracy of their measuring scale).

Lotter was one of the first to draw specific attention to the numerical imbalance between autistic girls and boys. Overall, there were over twice as many boys as girls (2.6:1) among those children deemed autistic. It is worth reminding ourselves that there would have been a high level of subjectivity as to the assessment of the 'behavioural peculiarities' that formed the basis of the original referrals. A recurrent theme in discussions of such assessments is that teachers or school officials are more inclined to view boys' behaviour as problematic than girls', so this could have been a factor. Lotter noted that the imbalance in his finding was lower than the male-female imbalance Kanner had reported earlier, but offered no explanation. In a more profoundly affected subgroup of fifteen children, the boy:girl ratio was 2.75:1. Classifying the cases by IQ, all of those with IQs above fifty-five were boys. Where were the girls? Lotter admitted their absence was puzzling but had no answer.

So, at the beginning of the 60s, autism was still viewed as a relatively rare and quite severe problem, although calculations as to its incidence were somewhat haphazard. A preponderance of boys was emerging as a consistent theme, but there had been no comment as to why this might be or whether the girls presented differently from the boys.

In the early 1980s came Wing and Gould's 'triad of impairments', a widening definition of autism in DSM-4, and the inclusion of Asperger's syndrome.[21] Together with greater public awareness of autism, the changes in diagnostic criteria and the inclusion of milder forms of the condition resulted in a dramatic increase in numbers, sufficient to raise concerns about an epidemic. Male-to-female ratios seemed to remain fairly stable, of the order of about four to one – higher than Lotter's assessment but relatively consistent across the various prevalence reports that were coming in. The inclusion of Asperger's syndrome raised the profile of the maleness of autism, and Lorna Wing frequently drew attention to Asperger's stance on this (at this point obviously unaware of the potentially sinister background to his findings). In one (much-quoted) study, she reported a male:female ratio of 15:1 in Asperger-type cases, which did much to back up the autism-as-a-male-problem story.[22]

But these more extreme figures were often not replicated. In Sweden, a total population study of Asperger's syndrome by psychologists Stephan Ehlers and Christopher Gillberg in 1993 revealed a prevalence of 3.6 per 10,000 children, with a male: female ratio of 4:1, echoing Kanner's original estimate.[23] In 2021, a study from Norway, sampling over two million adults and children, reported a male:female ratio of 3.67:1 in children and 2.57:1 in adults.[24] The authors suggested that the decrease in adults might reflect later diagnoses in females or diagnostic biases.

In 2017, a UK team headed by Rachel Loomes, a clinical psychologist, carried out a systematic review and meta-analysis of autism prevalence studies, specifically looking into the male-to-female ratio.[25] They considered issues such as whether or not a survey used active screening, which is when a general population was surveyed to try to identify all cases regardless of whether there had already been a diagnosis (as in Lotter's study mentioned previously). The alternative was passive screening, where only those who had already been diagnosed were counted. Looking at fifty-four studies, the overall 4:1 male:female ratio seemed to be confirmed. But the authors pointed out that there was considerable variability in the methods and findings of the different studies. In particular they noted that studies using active screening techniques were more likely to come up with lower ratios, of the order of about 3.25:1, whereas passive techniques were associated with ratios of about 5.5:1. They raised the issue of whether or not the screening tests being used might be more likely to miss females. They did not follow up on this question, but it planted a seed that later bore fruit. The authors still felt that the numbers suggested that boys were more likely to be diagnosed with autism than girls.

Eric Fombonne, a French-Canadian psychiatrist, has published widely on the issue of autism prevalence and the associated male:female ratios, as well as the increase in rates of diagnosis. In 2022, he reviewed 141 epidemiological surveys of autism from thirty-seven countries published since 1966. He reported that the male:female ratio (4.1:1) had remained stable over time.[26]

The numbers, although quite varied, do seem to provide firm evidence for the notion that autism is a predominantly male condition, sufficiently reliable that maleness could or even should be considered a defining characteristic. But remember these statistics mostly involve passive screening, and reflect the rates of diagnosis. It is difficult to access the rates at which problems might be flagged by families or carers, or by health care professionals or teachers, or the rates at which such concerns are translated into referrals for assessment. And then, of course, the rates at which such referrals result in a diagnosis of autism. Are we sure that concerns about possible autism are the same for girls and boys? Are we sure that girls and boys have equal access to assessment sessions, and are we sure that the tests used are even-handed when it comes to measuring differences in girls as opposed to differences in boys? Could autism's male spotlight at these 'entry points' into autism statistics be skewing the data?

GETTING PAST THE DOOR

There is clear evidence that it is much harder for girls to be referred for an autism assessment than for boys. In 2021, a team from the Institute of Psychiatry and Birkbeck College, both in London, surveyed the kinds of barriers that prevent or delay girls from getting a diagnosis.[27] They found that boys are referred for a diagnostic assessment ten times more often than girls. Moreover, where an assessment had been requested it took much longer for girls to get an appointment, sometimes as much as two years longer.

You might think that this is just a reflection of the numbers showing that more boys than girls are on the spectrum. In 2012, Professor Ginny Russell from University of Exeter, in an ongoing longitudinal study, investigated children who, even though they showed marked signs of autistic traits, had not been referred for diagnosis, and compared them to children who *had* been diagnosed.[28] It turned out that there were significantly more girls in the undiagnosed group, among them girls who showed symptoms just as severe as those shown by boys who had been diagnosed.

In other, more qualitative studies, parents of autistic daughters reported the difficulties they had in getting an assessment, of being disregarded by medical professionals, who used phrases such as 'late bloomer' or 'just shy' to describe their daughters. Page Pelphrey, the wife of autism researcher Kevin Pelphrey, referred to earlier, whose daughter Frances is autistic (as well as her son, Lowell), tells of how hard it was to get a diagnosis for their daughter. She reported that they 'went from doctor to doctor and were told to simply watch and wait . . . We got a lot of different random little diagnoses', she recalls. 'They kept saying, "Oh, you have a girl. It's not autism."'[29] Another study reported that parental beliefs about autism could also stand in the way of a timely diagnosis, with parents almost twice as likely to raise concerns about autism for boys than for girls.[30]

Teachers are often gatekeepers to autism assessments. Aware of the differences they see daily in the classroom, they may be the first to identify differences as difficulties, and to flag up the need for more in-depth observation and assessment. So might we find a male spotlight problem in the education profession too? A study in 2020 by some of the key players in the study of girls and women on the spectrum found that, as they politely put it, 'primary school educators might need extra help to improve the recognition of girls on the autism spectrum'.[31] They presented 289 teachers and teaching assistants with written vignettes describing girls and boys with various unusual behavioural characteristics. These might include descriptions such as 'Tries to join in with the other children but tends to be ignored', or 'If there is any free time in the classroom, . . . will spend it playing with Harry Potter cards'. The teachers were asked to rate the likelihood that the child – either 'Jack' or 'Chloe' – that they were reading about was autistic, as well as the likelihood that they would seek help for the child. As the researchers had predicted, Jack was much more likely to be identified as autistic and in need of help, as opposed to Chloe, even when the descriptions of their problems were identical.

It is clear that the road to diagnosis is not the same for females and males. And, once girls get as far as an assessment, it turns out that the tests themselves can serve as an additional barrier.

TESTING THE TESTS

We have already encountered autism's so-called gold standard tests, commonly a combination of ADOS and ADI tests. We know they can include rather ill-defined questions about behaviours being 'abnormal' or 'unusual', with the phrases 'for a boy' or 'for a girl' carefully excluded. What about the norms, those numerical thresholds above which you might be deemed atypical? These are developed by testing the sensitivity of the test (how good it is at correctly identifying those with autism) and the specificity (how good it is at correctly identifying those without). However, because the test is benchmarked against diagnosed populations, any biases that already exist are baked in. If you test the tests against already diagnosed populations, where there are more boys than girls, then it will be the patterns of behaviour seen in boys that will determine the clinical thresholds. Additionally, if there are very few girls, then it would be difficult to identify some kind of norm against which to measure them. Effectively, this means that you cannot have gendered norms in such tests. Male or female, all those taking the test will be measured against the same norms of 'usual' or 'unusual', 'normal' or 'abnormal'. A clinician might pat herself on the back for using gender-neutral tests. But if autism does not present in the same way in girls as in boys, then girls will not be correctly identified, and are more likely to be incorrectly excluded.

A multicentre Dutch study published in 2017 reported on all child referrals to one of six mental health services between 2011 and 2012.[32] A range of difficulties, including social/relationship problems, hyperactivity/concentration problems, anxiety/mood problems, and cognitive problems had been identified by parents, general practitioners, or other healthcare workers. Over twelve hundred children were screened, and 310 boys (35 per cent of the 885 boys referred) and 118 girls (30 per cent of the 396 girls referred) were identified as fulfilling the criteria for a diagnosis of autism. So, at this stage, the percentages of referred boys and girls identified as at risk for autism were roughly the same. All were then offered a full autism assessment. There were some dropouts who didn't complete this stage, leaving 121 boys and 49 girls to be tested. Of these, 86 boys (71 per cent of the tested cohort) and 23 girls (47 per cent of the tested cohort) received a confirmed diagnosis of autism. Boys, then, were 2.18 times as likely to receive an autism diagnosis than girls, even though about the same percentage of girls as boys had initially been identified as giving cause for concern.

The authors looked for what might have tipped the balance. Girls with more emotional or 'acting out' problems were more likely to be identified as autistic than other girls, meaning that those who were more withdrawn ('shy') or compliant ('good girls') were being screened out. Additionally, girls achieved lower scores than boys on measures of repetitive behaviours and highly focussed special interests. This would also have 'moved the needle' away from an autism diagnosis. The conclusion was that there was a strong probability that girls were being under-identified by the autism screening process, or 'not adequately captured by current instruments'.

Are we missing females just because autism detectors are not calibrated sufficiently sensitively for them? Whether or not the 'gold standard' autism assessment systems (in their current versions of ADOS-2 and ADI-R) are fit for purpose when they appear to miss so many cases has become something of a hot topic in both clinical and research fields. One call has been to introduce sex-specific scoring, suggesting different thresholds for females and males. Or to provide more detailed individual profiles based on the different constituent parts of the test that together contribute to a single score. Does someone initially present with appropriate social conversation, but then turn out to be speaking to a fairly rigid script? Is someone apparently good at making friends but struggles to keep them? Historically, individual datasets in different surveys or studies have generally been quite small, and, of course, the numbers of females within those datasets even smaller. As a result, it has proved hard to get sufficient numbers to investigate more nuanced impressions of different presentations of autism-based behavioural differences.

A recent large-scale survey claimed to have solved this problem by combining data from eight different autism networks, comprising twenty-seven separate sites, giving them access to nearly nine thousand 'confirmed' cases.[33] So far, so good, perhaps. But a glance at the demographics of this great sample revealed that 84 per cent of them were male. This feels like being back to the same vicious cycle. No comment on this imbalance was made in the paper, other than a slightly self-congratulatory note that the 1,463 girls who did make it into the study comprised a 'very large sample'.

The question asked of this dataset was whether diagnosed females were different from diagnosed males and, if so, how. But, besides the gender bias, there was also the recurrent problem that, if these autistic females have passed a clinical threshold that has been determined by measurements mainly based on autistic males, then they will invariably be quite like males. This proved to be the case. The authors reported 'minimal differences due to sex', apart from younger girls receiving (minimally) 'less severe' scores on 'repetitive and restricted behaviour', and adolescent girls, again minimally, receiving more severe scores on social responsiveness measures. There was a caveat that perhaps some girls might exhibit '*different* [author emphasis] ASD-related difficulties'. But of course, the measurement tools weren't calibrated to pick these up. The impression given by this paper was that the assessment tools were fit for purpose, and the fact that they identified fewer females was because the females didn't make the diagnostic cut, not that the females didn't make the diagnostic cut because the assessment tools were *not* fit for purpose.

Allison Ratto of the Children's National Hospital in Washington, DC, published an admirably polite commentary on the study.[34] She noted that the diagnostic tools used were based on male-dominated samples but also went further to point out an even wider problem of bias in all autism research to date:

> Most published research in autism uses fairly homogeneous samples, dominated by White, presumed cisgender and heterosexual males, usually residing in North America or Western Europe, most often from middle-class to upper-class socioeconomic backgrounds, who meet narrow criteria on specific gold standard measures.

So, while the tests were the gold standard, maybe that was true only for the select few. She called for the next stage in understanding autism to involve the autistic community itself, so that their insights could inform the questions that should be being asked.

An intriguing mathematical modelling study in Australia carried out a forecasting-type study to estimate sex differences in the 'hit rates' for autism diagnoses.[35] Data from nearly two thousand children between one and eighteen years of age who had been referred to a psychology clinic for assessment were used to estimate the probability of boys being diagnosed with autism as compared to girls. These probabilities were then 'weighted' by factors that had been shown to affect diagnoses in females as opposed to males. This included the so-called recognition bias – i.e., would a clinician even think that a troubled girl might be autistic? And then there was a diagnostic bias, the rate at which the diagnostic process was likely to find a girl autistic as opposed to a boy. Applying this biasing model to the clinical data revealed that as many as 80 per cent of the females might not have received an initial diagnosis of autism. As the author of the study, a clinician, points out, these 'missed' females can then be exposed to an 'alphabet soup of diagnoses', including depression, generalized anxiety disorder, social anxiety disorder, borderline personality disorder, bipolar disorder, and eating disorders.

It would seem that, even if somebody somewhere manages to make the case that a girl might be autistic, and gets her as far as the clinician's door, it does not mean that she will get through it.

AUTISM RESEARCH'S LEAKY PIPELINE

This 'gatekeeping' problem appears in the research world as well. If you are researching any kind of condition, you need to be sure that the participants in your research group do actually have it. You need to use reliable and valid tests of this condition – indeed, your research funding may well depend on it. This means that, in the autism research world, you will face what has been referred to as the 'cold, dead hand of ADOS'. In other words, you will be required to use autism's gold standard tests to confirm that your participants are genuinely autistic. This means that many females may be excluded from your research programme as they won't pass the gold standard threshold; those who do pass this threshold will, by definition, be pretty similar to males. So your sample may well be both biased and unbalanced.

This is called the 'leaky recruitment-to-research pipeline' problem. Even where recruitment and screening are population wide, and a potential pool of participants has been identified, for example by the use of autistic trait questionnaires (a so-called community diagnosis), researchers may then be required to use ADOS and/or ADI tests to select their final cohorts. A recent study from a group at MIT demonstrated that this can result in the exclusion of females at a rate over 2.5 times higher than males.[36] ADOS assessment tests were retrospectively applied to 145 adults whose autism had been indicated via a community diagnosis. After ADOS administration, twenty-five of the community-diagnosed females (50 per cent of the original cohort) were excluded from further research participation, compared with only 19 per cent of the males. This shifted the male:female ratio from 1.9:1 to 3.1:1 in the final research sample.

The leaky pipeline also affected a recent move towards encouraging autism research centres to come together and combine their datasets in order to increase the scale of autism studies. In my area, neuroimaging, the Autism Brain Imaging Data Exchange (ABIDE) was launched in 2012, aiming to facilitate the sharing of resting-state functional magnetic resonance imaging (fMRI) data from individuals with autism.[37] (This involves lying as motionless as possible in a scanner and staying awake but thinking of nothing – much harder than you might imagine!) In the first version of this initiative, ABIDE I, there were over a thousand fMRI resting-state datasets, as well as autism assessment data, from over 539 diagnosed autistic individuals. If you look closely at the numbers, you will find that 88 per cent of the datasets were from male participants, with 25 per cent of the sites invited to participate excluding females by design.

And here we encounter the 'cold, dead hand problem' again. One aspect of these autism datasets is that eligibility for inclusion almost invariably involves confirmation via the use of the gold standard ADOS and/or ADI tests. The MIT group that had revealed the consequences for their own dataset of this practice also surveyed several large publicly available autism datasets besides ABIDE II. They found that where ADOS had been used to determine inclusion, the male:female ratio was of the order of 7:1. Where the datasets used community diagnoses, the ratios varied from 0.68 to 1.8 to 1. It is perhaps unsurprising that a survey in 2021 of over 1,400 studies of brain-imaging research in autism showed that over 30 per cent of the studies were carried out on male-only groups. But more on that later!

We are, of course, getting into the realms of self-fulfilling prophecy. Picture the problem. The pool of potential participants that you might draw on for your research is primarily male, due to the barriers we've already discussed, with a handful of 'exceptional' females somehow making the cut. Then a second application of the fierce filtering system that has already screened out many of your possible female participants winnows out those remaining few at a rate twice that at which it is discarding males. As a researcher rather than a clinician, you might just accept this as the outcome of autism being a 'male' thing. You do your research on an entirely, or mostly, male population, their autism reliably verified by gold standard tests, and report your findings as though they apply to the entire autism population. Which appears to be characteristically male! And the findings of this research then inform the next updates of diagnostic criteria and tests.

The male spotlight problem has not only affected the practice of autism research; it has had a powerful influence on the theories behind it.

A MALE SPOTLIGHT CASE STUDY: THE EXTREME MALE BRAIN

A controversial hypothesis called the 'extreme male brain theory' was originally proposed in 2002 by the well-known psychologist Simon Baron-Cohen, head of the Autism Research Centre in Cambridge.[38] It is a theory that has had a long-lasting impact on the understanding of autism. Indeed, in another form of self-fulfilling prophecy, as a theory arising from a belief that autism is primarily a male problem, it has contributed significantly to continuing the belief that autism is primarily a male problem.

The extreme male brain theory involves a range of 'male-based' assumptions, and a certain amount of retrofitting of potential explanations about the condition. These assumptions include the following: In the typically developing population, there is such a thing as a biologically determined male brain that is, on average, reliably distinguishable from a female brain; these male brains can then be causally linked to specific aspects of male behaviour that, in turn, can reliably be distinguished from specific aspects of female behaviour. Digging a bit deeper, we find that, with respect to brains, their maleness can be causally linked to higher levels of prenatal testosterone. With respect to behaviour, males are, on average, supposedly better than females at understanding rule-based, abstract systems. Therefore, the maleness of a brain is linked to its prenatal hormonal marinade, resulting in the owner being more likely to be a 'systemizer'.

As we know, there is an assumption that autism is primarily a male condition. Therefore, following the thread in typical populations outlined previously, most autistic people will have male brains, so most autistic people will primarily be systemizers. You could, of course, work this chain of argument backwards – most autistic people show some kind of systemizing behaviour, so this could be linked to a male brain. At a more detailed level, as autistic behaviour is at the extreme end of systemizing behaviour, autistic individuals must have extreme male brains. In turn, the possession of such a brain could be linked to extreme levels of prenatal testosterone.

At the heart, then, of this somewhat tangled web is the assertion that autism is best understood through a male lens, as an atypical expression of extremely male (systemizing) behaviour linked to an extreme (male) brain. This lens has been calibrated by a wider set of assumptions about alleged differences between the brains of females and the brains of males (and just how big those differences might be), where those differences might come from, and what those differences might mean for the behaviours of the brains' owners. Does a particular type of brain make you more of a systemizer than an empathizer, for example, or more highly tuned to the demands of social situations?

The wider argument about 'male' and 'female' brains has been raging for a couple of centuries, and is still very much ongoing. In 2021, Lise Eliot of Rosalind Franklin University in Chicago and her team summarized thirty or so years of brain-imaging research and concluded that there was little or no reliable or consistent evidence that the brains of human males are somehow distinct from those of human females.[39] Her report cheerily urges us to 'dump the dimorphism', declaring that you can't 'sex' a brain. In addition, work by Daphna Joel at Tel Aviv University suggests that human brains are actually almost unique mosaics of characteristics that can be found in either male or female brains, so knowing whether someone is male or female will not tell you much about what their brain will look like.[40] But the 'hunt the difference' crusade rumbles on, now harnessing AI to find ways of proving that female brains can be distinguished from male brains. There are regular reports of new, ever more microscopic brain measurement techniques, with petabytes of painstakingly collected data being fed into highly sophisticated machine-learning programs to test whether the sex of brain ownership can be established. But we must remember that such studies are still, almost invariably, measuring only the size or strength of different structures.

We should also remember that many of these 'hunt the difference' quests have also ignored something we have only really been aware of for the last thirty years or so, and that is that our brains keep on changing throughout our adult lives, not just through our early years. This so-called 'neuroplasticity' should always be factored into any conclusions reached when brain differences are found between females and males. Does the brain of a female encounter the same world as the brain of a male? Will their respective owners play with the same toys, be exposed to the same social expectations, be treated in the same way by their parents or teachers, see identical representations of themselves in books and films and video games and on social media? Will they have the same experiences and training opportunities? If not, might this change their brains? The answer is almost definitely yes. Musicians, Tetris players, trainee jugglers, and taxi drivers have all found themselves in brain scanners to see how their particular talent might be reflected in brain changes, before, during, and after they acquired their specific skill. It is reflected quite clearly – did you know you can tell the difference between the brain of a keyboard player (symmetrical use of the hands reflected in the brain's motor cortex) and a string player (asymmetrical use of the hands)?

Any brain differences we find are not just a question of anatomy. What we really need to know is what such differences mean in how these owners experience the world, what they can achieve, and why, in some cases, things can go wrong.

So let's have a look at behaviour. Are males more likely to be systemizers? The idea of distinct and fixed sex differences in the full gamut of human behaviour has as long a history as that of beliefs about brains, and informs many sex/gender stereotypes. But, with respect to typical behaviour, there appears to be virtually no aspect of behaviour that you could guarantee as only (or even mainly) shown by males or only (or even mainly) females. Again, researchers have heroically trawled through many decades of psychology research and come up with much the same answer as the one about brains – there is little or no robust or consistent evidence that the behaviour of human males is somehow reliably distinct from that of human females. To paraphrase another firm statement from such researchers, 'Men are not from Mars or women from Venus. We are all from Earth'. This may well cue an outraged readers' list about men not being able to find anything in the fridge or women being the ones to remember birthdays but, trust me, I've done the numbers![41]

If we should discard the notion of a typical male brain and a typical set of male skills, where does this leave the extreme male brain theory? We should, perhaps, acknowledge that we are talking about *atypical* brains and behaviour and see if the chain of argument plays out better there.

With respect to brains and the *causal* role of prenatal or foetal testosterone in generating an autistic brain, the evidence is often indirect and, overall, inconclusive. As you might suppose, it is not straightforward to measure hormone levels in developing human foetuses, and the chosen metric, looking at such levels in fluid collected via amniocentesis, has not been universally accepted as a reliable measure. And there have been no consistent findings linking variations in prenatal testosterone to variations in specific brain structures in autistic individuals. But even if there were, the jury is still out on the exact links between structure and function in the human brain.

With respect to characterizing autism as associated with atypically high levels of systemizing behaviour and low levels of empathy, this too has been challenged, within research circles where measures of these patterns of behaviour have been deemed questionable, although, as we shall see later, Baron-Cohen's team have collected vast swathes of data using such measures. At the population level, when comparing very large numbers of females and males, analyses of some of these data do reveal statistically significant differences, but they are characteristically small, and actually expose the tremendous variability within the two groups, with a tremendous overlap between them.[42]

We should note that a key problem with the extreme male brain theory is that of impression management. Clearly there are theoretical and methodological issues to be debated, but much of extreme male brain's bad press has been around what has been *inferred* from the various assumptions. For example, one criticism is that, with its emphasis on the maleness of the condition, the theory appears to overlook female and (more recently) non-binary autistic individuals. The autistic community also felt that the focus on one particular cognitive aspect of autism, systemizing, overlooked what were often more incapacitating aspects of the condition, such as high levels of anxiety or marked sensory sensitivities. In addition, there was a strong either-or impression that systemizing was heightened at the expense of empathizing, with the unwelcome inference that autistic individuals were unempathetic.

On a more general level, not exclusively focussed on autism, the presentation of the theory has been accused of reinforcing sexist stereotypes about 'essential' differences between females and males, in terms of both the kind of brain they have and the kinds of skills linked to these brains. The use of the term 'male brain' unsurprisingly allows non-experts (or even some experts) to assume that this must uniquely refer to the brains of men. Despite a rather tardy observation in Baron-Cohen's book *The Essential Difference*, that you do not have to be a male to have a male brain, this nuanced definition has rather got 'lost in translation'.[43]

This issue of impression management is not trivial in assessing the impact that scientific theories and practices can have on understanding a condition that affects so many individuals. As we will see throughout the course of this book, once a belief about a condition such as autism gets established in the public (and, indeed, the scientific) consciousness, it can skew efforts to understand the condition and also prove inordinately difficult to dislodge. This is key to one of my concerns about the ongoing emphasis on autism as a male problem, especially when it affects what research is done and how it gets reported. Quite often there is a disconnect between what is going on within the pages of research journals, and attempts to correct beliefs in the public domain about such theories, which have been sustained by once firmly asserted and popularized findings. When it turns out that such findings can be misleading, I think there should be concerted attempts to put the record straight. Hence my previous book against the notion of female and male brains. Stereotypes are powerful social and cultural influences, and can stand in the way of attempted progress towards a greater understanding of many aspects of the human condition, including autism.

More recently, Simon Baron-Cohen has dialled back somewhat his emphasis on male brains – extreme or otherwise. In his latest book, *The Pattern Seekers,* his focus is firmly on a logic-based, systemizing approach to the world, a characteristic product of the autistic mind, and how this form of information-processing has been the evolutionary basis of human progress and creativity.[44] He still makes reference to sex differences in discussions of the systemizing-empathizing profile and its presentation in autistic people, but much more in terms of potential influences rather than causes, and on the autistic mind rather than the autistic brain. His attention has shifted to the balance between empathizing-systemizing skills at the population level – so a spotlight instead on behavioural strengths and weaknesses and their relevance to autism. This is a rather more understandable focus when trying to understand a condition that is (currently) only identifiable by atypical behaviour.

Indeed, in a podcast in November 2020, Baron-Cohen withdrew his earlier assertions about male (and female) brains, stating it was time to 'publicly retract some of that language around male and female brains', and that we 'don't need to refer to gender anymore'.[45] (This might be news to a female acquaintance of mine who was told just last year that she was autistic because she had an extreme male brain. She wondered if that was supposed to be some kind of accolade. Or a consolation prize.)

Even though Baron-Cohen has retracted some of his original language, the extreme male brain theory has left its imprint. Sarah Richardson from Harvard's GenderSci Lab and her colleague Eva Gillis-Buck have pointed out that the apparently unquestioned acceptance of the basic precepts of the extreme male brain theory –

that brains and behaviour can be sexed, and that females and males can be sorted into discrete categories – has been associated with a major focus of research efforts and funding on finding the biological causes of such differences at all levels, not only in autism but also in the research arena of sex differences as a whole.[46] This is not to deny that biological sex is certainly relevant and influential, but to emphasize that we need to look beyond it to find answers to many key questions.

Now we've seen how the 'maleness' thread weaves through so many parts of the ongoing autism story. So many women have been excluded from the narrative, not only by the clinicians who might be able to help, but also by researchers who might be able to track the causes and consequences of the condition. As chapter 1 showed, it took quite a long and complicated journey to arrive at today's official description of what autism looks like, the so-called autism phenotype. But somehow women got left out en route. Could the problem be that autism actually looks different in women? It may not be that the diagnostic tests are just not very good at spotting them, but that the tests have been designed with a different 'kind' of autism in mind. In order to explore this idea, we need to find out whether autistic women are differently different.

CHAPTER 3

FEMALE AUTISM

DIFFERENTLY DIFFERENT?

Autism is a term applied to an extraordinarily wide range of unusual behaviours. Yet, despite the wide contemporary definition of autism and the extensive array of metrics, we are somehow managing to overlook a highly significant group who could and should be part of the autism story – women.

We don't miss them all, of course. Remember that Kanner did have three girls in his original group of eleven, and there always have been some girls in the various datasets that have accumulated over the years – but they are almost always in the vast minority. But the fact that early assertions of quite marked ratios of 15:1 or higher have now been revised to the more commonly accepted 4:1 or even – after a closer look – 2:1, shows that, for whatever reason, autistic females have always been harder to spot.

At this point, we should perhaps remind ourselves that when we are looking at the more profound type of autism, characterized by often severely disruptive patterns of behaviour and marked intellectual disability, there are roughly equal numbers of females and males – or, at least, the difference in the male: female ratio is much less marked. Is there any evidence here that the behavioural patterns are different in females? As someone who has spent time with more profoundly impaired autistic people, I know that assessments of any aspect of their behaviour can be very challenging – they are often nonverbal or minimally verbal, find it difficult to follow instructions, and are easily distracted or distressed. So it can be hard to make any general comments about patterns of behaviour. Although the profoundly impaired could be a better source for checking both the similarities and differences of autistic females and males, it is not an area much explored.

Some studies have found that females with profound autism may appear more eager to connect with other people and to seek out social interactions, despite having severe difficulties with social communication, whereas males with profound autism may be more likely to exhibit behaviours likely to harm themselves, such as headbanging, or have more severe impairments in adaptive functioning, such as daily living skills. But overall, there have been no consistent findings that might distinguish females from males at this end of the spectrum. It is possible that, in the future, a greater focus on differences between autistic females and males may shift towards those with more severe difficulties but, for the time being, most studies are focussed at the 'other end' of the spectrum, where the differences are more evident.

THE HUNT FOR THE DIFFERENCE AGENDA: WHY IS IT MISSING IN AUTISM?

In my previous book (and since), I protested loud and long against the centuries-old obsession with finding differences between both the brains and the behaviour of females and males. This has apparently 'outed' me as a 'sex difference denier' who, as such, is putting women's health at risk by calling for a ban on sex differences research. (I'm not, but it is apparently too good a 'straw man' to resist!) As I explained in the preface, there are well-documented sex differences between certain brain-related conditions that should indeed be investigated with sex differences as part of the research design – a higher proportion of women suffer from Alzheimer's disease and depression, for example. What about 'male' diseases? Well, the condition that is most often cited as one where a sex differences perspective in any research design should be near compulsory is autism. And yet, as we have seen in the last chapter, one thing that has characterized so much of the post-Kanner years is a *lack* of sex differences research.

Is this void because of the male spotlight effect we've already investigated? Or is it due to Grunya Sukhareva's early observations on autistic girls being overlooked or Asperger's firm assertions that he couldn't find any, establishing a stereotype that autism is a male problem? Have we missed the girls because we just haven't been looking for them? A belief in the 'maleness' of autism has primed both the clinical and the collective consciousness, the diagnostic dice have been loaded, and other names have been found for unusual female behaviour.

Perhaps we are missing females because autism detectors are not calibrated sufficiently sensitively for them. Females have the same sort of presentations, the same sort of unusual behavioural patterns, but they are somehow flying beneath the radar. Is the problem simply a quieter, more muffled presentation, a softly, softly factor?

Or is there genuinely a different kind of autism in females that isn't captured by the clinical expectations or test criteria, validated as they have been on populations of males? Should we be looking for a female autism phenotype, a properly detailed picture of what this kind of autism might look like? In more generic discussions of sex/gender differences, we have detailed lists asserting that men are like 'this' and women are like 'that'. In autism, discussions seem to be more along the lines of 'autistic males are like "this"' and 'autistic females – er – aren't'. Have we just missed the girls because we have been looking at the wrong things?

There are quite a few hurdles to overcome before we can begin answering these questions. Not least of which is coming to a better understanding of what being a woman with autism is actually like, of how autistic women experience the world, not only differently from neurotypical females and males, but also perhaps differently from autistic men as well.

Listening to the many personal histories of ASD women who were diagnosed late, the initial wrong turn is often signposted by confident statements such as 'You can't be autistic, you're female'; 'Girls don't get autism'; or 'You've got friends and make eye contact, you can't be autistic'. And these are often comments from clinicians themselves, not just from those whose expertise is derived from autism stereotypes or Hollywood movies. But for those females who do get past this barrier, does their autism present differently?

'FLYING BENEATH THE RADAR'

A long-standing claim is that, on average, while it has been accepted that females can and do display typical patterns of autistic behaviour, these tend to present less severely than they do in males. The social isolation is not so extreme, the unusual patterns of movement or tics are less pronounced, the language delays are less evident. So, the profiles may be similar, but the need for intervention and support is rated as lower. Are girls really less affected by their autism? Perhaps all patterns of unusual behaviour are more 'muted' in females on the spectrum.

Remember Sukhareva's comment that 'The general picture of schizoid psychopathies is paler in girls than in boys, and the schizoid peculiarities appear less marked. Also the percentage of schizoid psychopathies seem to be lower in girls'. And many of the contemporary studies focussing on autistic females do generally report that they have lower scores in the overall standard assessments.[1] We should remember that both the ADOS and ADI tests offer examples guiding the expectations of clinicians (Does the child initiate social interaction and share with others?) and interviewees (Does your child have unusually narrow and focussed interests?). And if the answer is 'maybe', 'not especially', or 'sometimes', it will be given a lower score than a 'yes, definitely'.

It is possible that this less visible or 'paler' form of autism is an example of what is called 'internalizing behaviour'. Perhaps whatever it is that leads to autism and how it presents itself is the same for both males and females, but females are more likely to 'muffle' their difficulties. Psychopathological symptoms (not just in autism) are frequently categorized into 'internalizing' and 'externalizing' behaviours.[2] Internalizing refers to an inwardly focussed response to distress. Individuals show high levels of guilt and self-criticism, blaming themselves for perceived inadequacies and failures, and they frequently show patterns of social withdrawal or self-harm. Internalizing is linked to specific types of mental health issues such as depression and social anxiety. Externalizing refers to 'acting out' types of behaviours, such as anger and aggression and hyperactivity, and is linked to conduct disorder, oppositional defiant disorder, attention deficit hyperactivity disorder (ADHD), and substance use disorders.

There are consistent reports that evidence of internalizing is much more common in female mental health problems, and externalizing more common with male problems.[3] We could certainly describe how autism seems to present in females as evidence of an internalizing process at work. Compare the quiet intensity of a girl lining up her collection of stuffed toys in height order with the noisy acting out of ritualized routines evident among some boys.

When, later, we come to talk about camouflaging or masking tactics in the autistic female population, these would seem to be the very embodiment of internalizing. We will see that the need not to be noticed is a theme that emerges strongly from the personal testimonies of late-diagnosed women. They report putting considerable effort into masking or camouflaging any signs of autism, especially their social difficulties, and hiding them from the outside world. On the surface, all appears calm, but the inner turmoil can be hugely self-destructive.

There is evidence of a link between the internalizing behaviour more common in females with mental health problems and the 'low-key' presentation of autism in females. A recent worldwide survey of clinical professionals (covering thirty-one different countries) reported autistic males as displaying more externalizing behaviours, with female symptoms clearly described as internalizing. One of the professionals remarked that females were at risk of going undetected due to 'a lesser degree of challenging behaviour'.[4]

Where might this 'quieter' version of autistic behaviour come from? One suggestion is that females have an innate drive, a biological imperative of some kind, to be social, to fit in, to internalize any distress, which can make the recognized signs of autism less evident. Or could it be that girls are exposed to specific socialization processes that train them to be compliant and conforming, to not 'act out' or rock the boat, to fly beneath the radar? Of course, it could also be an entanglement of the two – another version of the 'biological script playing out on a social stage'.

BORN TO BE 'MILD'?

> We're raising our girls to be perfect, and we're raising our boys to be brave.
>
> —Reshma Saujani, founder of Girls Who Code

There is good evidence that being social is an innate human skill. Tobias Grossmann, whose research focusses on early cognitive development, refers to human infants entering the world 'tuned to their social environment and readily prepared for social interaction'.[5] Recent evidence has demonstrated the amazing social awareness and social rule-seeking behaviour present from birth in almost all babies. For example, at birth, babies can distinguish sounds from their native language from those of other languages.[6] They will respond differently to words spoken in an emotional tone – happy or sad or fearful – than to the same words spoken in a neutral tone.[7]

Is this equally true of all babies, or are some more 'naturally' social than others? Early investigators hunted for evidence of female/male differences in social behaviour in babies, even newborns. There were claims that baby girls are better at imitating behaviour, at recognizing familiar faces, and at responding to different emotional expressions, which could be construed as an early talent for 'reading the room'.[8] This might be taken as the basis for greater awareness of appropriate social behaviour, with the imitation skills making the effective mimicking of others more of an inbuilt option for girls. But, to date, there are no consistent findings that newborn baby girls arrive better equipped in the social stakes than their newborn brothers.

However, if you track the emergence of skills that show that you are learning the tricks of the social trade, such as maintaining eye contact with people speaking to you, or 'sharing' their emotions – e.g., showing signs of distress when they are upset – then baby girls do seem to pick up on these quicker that boys. Where might this come from?

Within the first four months since birth, girls, on average, maintain eye contact four times longer than boys.[9] Researchers have suggested that this tendency relates to how their mothers interact with them. On average, mothers spend longer in face-to-face contact with their daughters (think pulling funny faces, sticking out their tongue, and so forth) than with their sons, with whom they have higher rates of rough-and-tumble play (knee-bouncing, rollover games) that involve less eye contact. One possibility is that parents and carers are responding to some kind of invisible signals being generated by their manipulative little charges, with the girls calling for face-to-face play and the boys wanting to be thrown around the place. But there is another explanation. In one series of studies, researchers 'cross-dressed' babies according to gender stereotypes and gave them names associated with the other gender.[10] Observers naive to a baby's sex were shown to react differently to them depending on whether they thought they were female or male. When people thought they were playing with baby boys, they enthusiastically bounced them up and down or offered them tractors or hammers to play with. In contrast, the baby girls were cuddled and spoken to gently and offered dolls or soft toys. So the differences in social training opportunities would not seem to be linked to some kind of biological imperative, but more to the gendered expectations of infants' social circles.

Gendered socialization is a powerful force to which babies are exposed right from the moment of birth (with those ghastly gender reveal parties demonstrating that biased expectations are firmly in place well before human babies actually arrive on this planet). Joyce Endendijk is a Dutch psychologist and associate professor in developmental psychopathology at Erasmus University Rotterdam. Her research focusses on the development of gender differences in childhood and adolescence, with an emphasis on socialization processes, gender stereotypes, and gender identity.[11] She refers to gender-differentiated parenting, where parents create gender-specific environments for children via the toys they buy, the activities they encourage, the behaviours they reward. What you might call the 'Who's a pretty girl?'/'Man up' divide. But we shouldn't heap all the blame on parents. A quick survey of twenty-first-century gender bombardment means we are looking at gender-differentiated just-about-everything. Marketing of toys and clothes; role models via films, video games, social media, and so on; gender gaps in everything from education and pay to business and politics all convey the clear message that females and males are inevitably and irretrievably different.[12]

There are many examples of gendered social 'tuning', where different standards and expectations for girls and boys seem to be in play, and these can include the belief that different levels of conformity and compliance will be expected. Girls are more often rewarded for socially appropriate behaviour, such as being polite, sitting still, being helpful, or joining in group play. 'Toys for girls' are therefore much more likely to encourage such group activities. And girls are more often chastised for socially inappropriate behaviours such as rowdiness, untidiness, or 'tomboyishness', which are all stereotypical of boys. As a result, girls have a greater awareness of the importance of social rules, conformity, and friendship networks. Behaviourally, there is evidence that, on average, girls are much more responsive to socialization pressures than boys are. For example, young girls' choices appear to be more easily moulded by any kind of signal that items such as toys or clothes or books or games are 'for girls'. Hence the power of pink.[13]

THE FEMALE EMPATHY STORY

Other claims concerning female superiority in social skills include emphatic assertions that females have an inbuilt advantage in one particular core social skill, namely the power of understanding others, of empathy. Empathy does, indeed, play a key role in the making of a sociable being (of any kind). If you are going to successfully connect with someone, you need to be able to recognize or understand their mental state: Are they happy, sad, angry, or bored? This emotion-detector system is referred to as the cognitive component of empathy. There is also an emotional component, which has more to do with insight into someone else's emotional state – responding to it with an appropriate emotion, the concept of 'sharing your pain'.[14] One of the most debated sex differences in human behaviour is the alleged female superiority in empathy.

Being empathic (however that comes about) is a skill that is stereotypically attributed more to women than to men – hence references to empathic female leadership (which, in certain instances, might stand as evidence of the unreliability of stereotypes!). The opening lines of Simon Baron-Cohen's book on sex differences asserted that 'the female brain is hard-wired for empathy'.[15] Evolutionarily informed theories propose that females *needed* to be more sociable and collaborative so they could secure membership into mutually protective networks – the 'safety in numbers' factor.

If females are naturally more empathic, then the expectation would be that sex differences in empathy might be present from a very early age. One measure of empathic behaviour in babies is the length of time they maintain eye contact with another person. As we have seen, there is no evidence of sex differences in very young infants, although there is evidence of a divergence by the age of about four months.

Could we again be looking at the consequence of social training? Is there any evidence that girls receive more empathy training than boys? It does appear that girls are often socialized to prioritize the needs and emotions of others and to be more sensitive to the feelings of those around them. One study published in the journal *Sex Roles* found that parents were more likely to use emotion-focussed language with their daughters, such as talking about emotions and feelings, compared to their sons.[16] Additionally, girls were more likely to be encouraged to express and share their emotions, while boys were more likely to be encouraged to regulate or suppress them.

The notion that females are more empathic than males also appears to be one of those self-fulfilling stereotypes. Much of the evidence around greater female empathy comes from self-report measures. But if researchers disguise the fact that they are assessing empathy, on the whole sex differences disappear. So there may be a strong element of living up to expectations. But, as we know, expectations can exert powerful influences on both brain and behaviour. If, from an early age, it is clear that you are expected to be nurturing or caring or emotionally sensitive, and it is frowned on if you are not, then, on the whole, this is how you will behave.

We have, of course, come across the notion of greater empathy in women in chapter 2 when discussing Simon Baron-Cohen's early accounts of his extreme male brain theory, where he claimed that understanding the emotions of others, or empathizing, was an innately brain-based feminine skill, as opposed to understanding systems, or systemizing, which was conversely an innately brain-based masculine skill. Nowadays, with respect to autism, Baron-Cohen has reduced his emphasis on biological maleness as the most important causal factor, but has gathered some powerful datasets measuring the empathizing-systemizing dimension in human behaviour.

One large-scale study, in 2018, took advantage of a television documentary on autism to gather data from more than half a million viewers, including more than 36,000 individuals identifying as autistic, who completed, among other questionnaires, the empathizing-systemizing scale.[17] As predicted, females had, on average, higher scores on the empathy quotient than males, although there was quite a degree of overlap between the two populations. A second study, in 2023, gathered six years' worth of data from over 300,000 people in fifty-seven different countries.[18] The test used was the 'Reading the Mind in the Eyes' Test (RMET), a paper-and-pencil test that can be run online. Respondents are shown an image of just the eye portion of the human face. (This was an unusual experience until the recent pandemic, when we suddenly found ourselves conversing with a world full of mask wearers.) Participants were asked to report which of four words best describes what the person in the picture is thinking or feeling, such as 'arrogant', 'sarcastic', 'grateful', or 'tentative'. Effectively, it is an emotion-recognition task. (You can try this yourself – google it.)

This enormous dataset revealed that if you looked at the female or male advantage in the test in each country, the results do make quite compelling reading: there was an average female advantage in thirty-six of the fifty-seven countries studied, with no countries showing male advantage. However, before we hail this as resounding support for the females-as-empathizers tale, we should note that within each of the countries studied, the average differences between females and males were actually what statisticians might call 'vanishingly small', with very little overall separation between the two groups. This is a cautionary note, rather than a full-on dismissal, but it does demonstrate that although sex differences may play a part in the autism-empathy story, many other factors should be considered too. There is, of course, the possibility that vanishingly small differences in a neurotypical population may play out differently in an autistic one, which is something we'll look at shortly. More recently, a meta-analysis of the RMET raised doubts as to whether it is really a valid measure of social cognitive ability.[19] So the jury is still out with respect to the role of empathy as a stand-alone female 'gift' that either moderates or disguises some of the emotional excesses of autism.

'I SHOULD JUST HAVE BURNT MORE CARS'

Part of our quest for autistic girls, then, has led us down the path of gendered socialization as the source of some form of behavioural restraint that is encouraged more in girls. Social constructivists would focus on the early training of girls to be well-behaved and socially sensitive. Feminist neuroscientists such as myself would point out the brain-changing effects of an undoubtedly gendered world. However we get there, there is evidence that females *are* more concerned about 'fitting in', about not being perceived as different, a powerful driving force in human behaviour. Could this force provide some kind of 'invisibility' cloak beneath which autistic girls may fly under the diagnostic radar?

Writing in 2012, social scientists Rebecca Jordan-Young and Keely Cheslack-Postava suggested that an environment of gendered socialization – the toys, clothes, role models, social media, etc. to which children are exposed – interacted with those biological processes that had increased a child's likelihood of developing autistic behaviour.[20] So whatever genetic factors set in motion, the many potential facets of an autism phenotype could be moulded by the world a child with an autistic brain encounters. Perhaps such differences in early social support training could dial down the more disconcerting presentations that might have initially caught the attention of parents and teachers, which would then underwhelm diagnosticians (with their own attitudes and expectations of what autism looks like). Cheslack-Postava and Jordan-Young refer to a 'pervasive developmental environment' where gender and its effects are critical ongoing pressures. Rather like our 'invisibility' cloak suggestion, they take a rather more positive view of the effects of female gender socialization, suggesting that it might serve as some kind of protective factor. They believe that female socialization may ameliorate the worst presentations of autistic behaviour and the stigma associated with 'acting different'.

There is a downside to such a disguise. One late-diagnosed autistic woman recounted how her quiet and passive behaviour had led to her autism going unnoticed for years and ruefully regretted that she had been so well-behaved: 'The reward for trying hard to be normal was to be ignored because you were acting normal and I look at stories online of kids who were going off the rails and I think, I should have just burnt more cars'.[21]

So far we have tracked the idea that for girls to be recognized as autistic, they must match up to a male prototype. Clinicians would be looking for evidence of social impairments and of RRBIs as in the male diagnostic profile. The impression we have been given is that some (few) girls will make the diagnostic cut, but often only just, as their presentation is generally milder.

The low numbers of girls that emerged from this one-size-fits-all approach has been taken as a measure of some form of biological protective effect that either makes girls less vulnerable (so they are less likely to 'get' autism) or will give rise to a symptom presentation that is less severe, so will not pass the diagnostic threshold. An additional hypothesis is that socialization training will cause the muffling or internalizing of autistic signs, serving as some kind of behavioural protective effect, again keeping girls flying beneath the radar. The conclusion has been that there *are* females on the spectrum but generally they are less socially impaired and less likely to display challenging RRBIs than diagnosed males.

ARE FEMALES MORE THAN JUST 'LESS' AUTISTIC?

But what we have been missing, with the spotlight firmly focussed on the autism-as-male notion, is a rather more nuanced discussion about whether or not, even within the two defining categories of autistic behaviour, there might be any fundamental differences between the girls who had been diagnosed as autistic and the boys. From a clinical point of view, such differences might provide clues as to what interventions might help (or not), or what kind of advice or prognoses you might be able to give to parents, carers, or autistic individuals themselves.

Back in 2011, there were fewer than ten studies directly comparing autistic females and males, beyond the almost incidental observations that autistic girls seemed less impaired than the boys. This is despite observations in the 1980s, by psychologists such as Lorna Wing and Judith Gould, that the lack of autistic females was something of a conundrum. A review in 2011 covered the findings to date and reported relatively few consistent findings in overall measures.[22] But at this stage, of course, the studies being reviewed were still a reflection of autism's male spotlight problem, resulting in a limited number of women with diagnoses based on potentially gender-biased instruments.

Atypical social behaviour is, and always has been, at the core of what constitutes autism. Recall Sukhareva's description of her children's 'failure to connect'. As we have seen, this characteristic is reflected worldwide, with deliberate social withdrawal captured in the different names for autism, such as the Japanese term *jheisyo* (intentionally shut). Difficulties with 'social communication and social interaction' is the overall term given to this key feature of autism. This is a fairly broad-brush concept. It covers understanding the rules of social behaviour such as turn-taking in conversation, respect of personal space, and monitoring of other people's responses and adapting behaviour accordingly. You also need to understand when to inhibit inappropriate behaviour and not commit social faux pas. There is a language aspect, too, as you may have to go beyond a literal understanding of what people are saying and consider things such as irony, sarcasm, jokes, and puns. Perhaps most of all, you need to be motivated to interact and communicate with other people: to be a social being.

Early investigations into autistic sex differences were, of course, based on diagnosed females, and as a result found few, if any, significant sex differences in the broadly construed sociability measures. It was not until subtypes of social behaviour were more closely assessed, and/or researchers spread their autism net more widely and incorporated population measures of autism, that sex differences started emerging.[23] Younger autistic girls were reportedly better at imitation and pretend play, and, in general, appeared to have better conversation skills. However, one clinician commented that when she met one young girl for a second time, the marked similarity to the wholly socially appropriate answers the child had given the first time she met her made her suspect that there was some kind of well-learned script at play.[24]

Several studies using special measures of social motivation, such as interest in socializing and forming relationships, revealed that autistic females were much more likely to understand this aspect of social behaviour and to be aware of social rules, such as not to invade personal space or to be prepared to join in on group activities. This information was elicited by talking to parents and carers and teachers, and focussed on everyday, natural settings. Beyond simple 'yes'/'no' answers it was also possible to provide some very telling context. For example, a question about whether or not a child has difficulty making friends might elicit a comment along the lines of 'yes' for a boy and 'no' for a girl. But behind these answers could be different subtexts. The 'yes' for a boy could be qualified by 'but he's not really interested in friends, he's always been a bit of a loner'. The 'no' for a girl could be qualified by 'but she seems to have difficulties hanging on to friends, and may land up with just one or two that she's very clingy about, and then they seem to fall out'.[25]

Once there was a critical mass of studies looking at more detailed aspects of the broad-brush concepts measured by full-blown autism diagnoses, it was possible to do a large-scale survey of the findings to see if any consistent patterns were emerging. One such survey was carried out in 2021 by Henry Wood-Downie, a UK psychologist, and colleagues.[26] Initial scrutiny of the literature revealed over seven hundred relevant studies since 2003, which shows how interest in this topic has, pleasingly, escalated. They weeded out those of poor quality or with small samples or inadequate assessments of autism (they excluded studies where ADOS and ADI were the only assessments used) and, particularly, those that didn't include both autistic and neurotypical males and females. Across the sixteen selected studies, a consistent message emerged: autistic females had significantly better social interaction and social communication skills than autistic males. This sex difference was also shown in non-autistic groups, with non-autistic females showing superior social skills compared to non-autistic males. Both autistic females and males were worse at social tasks than their non-autistic counterparts, and measures of social interaction and communication skills in non-autistic males were slightly better than in autistic females but this was not statistically significant.

The authors felt that the lack of such clear-cut findings in earlier studies was possibly related to a reliance on the kind of global scores that the standard assessments provided, and the real differences were only emerging with more detailed profiling. So, with respect to 'difficulties with social interaction', we are starting to get a picture of specific aspects of social behaviour that distinguish autistic females from autistic males.

EMPATHY IN FEMALE AUTISM

The role of empathy has been a consistent thread through the autism story, from Kanner, for example, noting his children's lack of affective contact, through to 1980s models suggesting that autistic individuals suffered from a kind of 'mindblindness', a lack of empathy, an inability to 'read' other people's emotions or to infer what they might be feeling from the way they were behaving or the facial expressions they were displaying.[27] This lack of such an ability is obviously core to the empathizing-systemizing dimension in Baron-Cohen's conceptualization of autistic behaviour at the beginning of this century, which we encountered in the last chapter. Now personal stories and newer research results indicate that differences in this aspect of social behaviour may provide a useful cue in tracking down autism's missing girls.

As we saw earlier, stereotypically, empathy has been linked more commonly to women than men, although we are beginning to acknowledge that the evidence in the neurotypical population is weak. What about in those with autism? Certainly there have been early studies reporting that ASD individuals (of either sex) score lower on questionnaire measures of empathy than non-ASD peers. If empathy is a trait more common in females than males, do autistic females show more empathy than autistic males, even if both groups show less evidence of empathy overall? The initial answer appeared to be no, as most early research found no sex differences in self-report measures of empathy in autistic groups.[28] Could this be another one for the 'autistic females are like autistic males' dossier?

We need to remember that there is more than one aspect to empathy. There is the affective component, which refers to an ability to recognize and share someone else's emotions, and there is the cognitive component, which involves an assessment of the emotions you are seeing in someone else, and a decision as to how you might respond. A distinction you might describe as 'understanding from within' as opposed to 'understanding from without'.[29]

These components are neatly illustrated by a study looking at the responses of both autistic boys and girls to a contrived scenario in which the experimenter traps her finger in a ring binder.[30] Autistic girls were more likely to show 'emotion-focussed' responses ('Ooh, I bet that hurts'; 'Are you alright?') whereas boys were more 'problem-focussed' ('You should be more careful'; 'I can get you a bandage'). It was a small study (sixteen autistic girls and fifty-three autistic boys), with all participants assessed according to DSM-5 criteria, but it gave another indication that a closer look at apparently similar scores might reveal some intriguing differences.

With respect to understanding autism, it turns out that close attention to separate components of empathy is a very important distinction. It was not made in early discussions of autism and the impression given was that autism could be characterized as a general empathy deficit. This most certainly did not accord with the autism self-advocacy community, who reported that, quite often, they have a problem with too much empathy. Take this account by Amy, a mother of a twelve-year-old autistic girl:

> Jenni is like an emotional tuning-fork, turned up to the max if you know what I mean. If she sees something sad on the television she can become completely beside herself, crying and crying and inconsolable. Even if it is about something in a country a million miles away or that happened hundreds of years ago. We had a near escape with a film called *Old Yeller* which someone suggested Jenni might like to watch as she adores dogs. Luckily I found out about the sad ending – she'd probably still be crying.

Amy's description of Jenni would suggest that empathy 'deficits' in some autistic individuals may be more closely associated with the cognitive component of autism – you might be good at recognizing how someone was feeling but poor at understanding what to do about it. Fifteen-year-old Kayleigh reflected on her own struggles with behaving empathically:

> I could understand why people might be sad – if they'd broken up with their best friend or their dog had died. I could watch them being sad and feel really sad for them. And I could watch how other people made them feel better. But I could never work out how I could do that – not

> even how to make my face look right – so I would just walk away and then it looked like I didn't care.

Simon Baron-Cohen and his team have recently re-examined empathizing-systemizing issues in autism, devising a new measure – empathic disequilibrium.[31] Empathic disequilibrium refers to an imbalance between emotional and cognitive empathy. Studying a very large sample of both autistic and typical individuals, they found that a tendency towards higher emotional than cognitive empathy was linked both to diagnosed autism and to higher levels of autistic traits in the typical populations. And this empathic disequilibrium was much more prominent in autistic females. So a more nuanced measure of empathy is nicely matching the stories that autistic women are telling, and also indicating the advantages of looking beneath the surface.

The take-home message from this part of the discussion is that, although autistic girls did show higher levels of social skills than autistic boys in many aspects of social behaviour, they were still generally less socially able than non-autistic girls. This finding is supported by studies such as that by Felicity Sedgewick and colleagues from University College London, looking at friendship behaviour in autistic and neurotypical adolescents.[32] On the surface, the self-report experiences of autistic girls suggested they were similar to those of neurotypical girls (and more positive than those of autistic boys). But closer questioning revealed that the autistic girls had many more challenges maintaining their friendships and were often exposed to bullying within their friendship groups. Although this bias within autistic populations might mirror that which can be found at a population level in neurotypical populations, we should remember that, for autistic females, it is in the context of the other struggles that autism can bring. Being more socially sensitive and socially aware in a world in which you are different or not welcome might not always be beneficial. It might just sharpen any social rejection that you face.

ARE RRBIS REALLY RARE IN AUTISTIC FEMALES?

The other defining aspect of autism (as a whole) is that of RRBIs.[33] Early research into RRBIs almost invariably reported that they were rare in diagnosed girls, or less marked. Looking at specific diagnostic criteria, this was especially true of 'circumscribed interests' and 'unusual preoccupations' – but remember we have already noted that there are no gendered norms for what counts as 'unusual' or 'circumscribed'. And, of course, these studies, although large scale, are looking at women who have managed to pass the diagnostic threshold, not those who haven't.

However, the emergence of a specific questionnaire related to RRBIs – the Bodfish Repetitive Behavior Scale–Revised – published in 1999 started to throw more detailed light on these specific behaviours.[34] This particular questionnaire includes forty-three items in all, with answers scaled from 0 (no occurrence) to 4 (high frequency and intensity). Questions include whether or not the person being assessed has specific routines and rituals that have to be followed every day, or unusual attachments to certain objects, or tendencies to injure themselves by headbanging or biting or hair or skin pulling.

A study in 2019 by Ligia Antezana and colleagues took a closer look at RRBIs in girls.[35] They examined scores on each of the forty-three items on the Bodfish scale. They found different types of behaviour were more common in girls, such as hair pulling and skin picking, forming strong attachment to single objects, and passionate insistence on sameness (such as sitting in the same place). Autistic boys were more likely to engage in repetitive self-stimulatory behaviours, such as rocking, flapping, and spinning.

These self-stimulatory behaviours are known as 'stimming' and can be one of the most disconcerting aspects of how autism presents to other people, as they can clearly set an individual apart from everyday patterns of typical behaviour. They are reportedly less evident in girls, and it has been suggested that this might be the distinguishing characteristic between autistic females and males. But, particularly if you focus on the lived experience testimonies of autistic females, this difference may not be because girls do not engage in 'stimming' behaviours but because they make enormous efforts to hide them. The science journalist Sue Nelson, writing about her discovery, at the age of sixty, that she is autistic, remembered that, as a child, she found 'swirling and gentle rocking mesmerizingly soothing', and then added that, as an adult, she still body rocks occasionally 'though only ever in private, because I know it makes most observers uncomfortable'.[36]

The issue of the social acceptance (or not) of stimming was raised in a series of interviews with autistic adults in 2019.[37] As well as a near-universal assertion that they used stimming as a calming or soothing mechanism, the hunt for socially acceptable alternatives or ways of concealing stimming was a common theme. One woman reported tapping rhythmically on her leg rather than on her desk, another of shutting herself in the safe space of her car. The powerful drive to try and disguise a soothing ritual in order not to make other people feel uncomfortable is something of a 'double whammy' for autistic females, often urgently anxious not to be marked out as different or weird. Again, we see a surface assessment resulting in 'minimally present' with respect to the occurrence of RRBIs in females, which fails to give the full picture.

Once a critical mass of studies specifically addressing the issue of RRBIs and their role in determining whether or not females get a diagnosis had been carried out, it was possible to undertake systematic surveys of the findings. A paper in 2020 showed that RRBI scores were indeed a significant factor in differential female/male diagnosis.[38] Because RRBIs were considered more characteristic of males on the spectrum, greater attention was paid to this aspect of behaviour when boys were being diagnosed. Where RRBIs were noted in girls, less diagnostic significance was attached to them. This was particularly true when it came to the 'restricted interests' part of RRBIs, where there was evidence of an inbuilt male bias in the assessment of what was deemed 'restricted'.

What happened when researchers drilled down into autistic patterns of behaviour and asked detailed questions about girls as well as boys? It began to look as if females did, indeed, have their own kind of highly focussed interests, but they weren't on the 'approved' list of weather patterns or transport systems or mathematical calculations listed in the diagnostic tests. Parents might be quizzed about their son's obsession with dinosaurs or car badges but not about their daughter's highly focussed interest in, say, Barbie dolls or Hello Kitty items or stuffed toys. All girls are interested in these things, right? Nothing to see here! A possible warning sign was being overlooked.

Tony Attwood is a British psychologist now working in Australia. He was one of the first researchers to focus on autism in girls, an extension of his earlier work on Asperger's syndrome. He noted this RRBI problem, that autistic girls may have different kinds of 'special interests' than boys.[39] These could appear typical (or, indeed, stereotypical) on the surface, but closer inspection might reveal a highly focussed fascination, such as gathering all known facts about show ponies or boy bands or Barbie, or a rigid insistence on routines around riding or grooming. Compulsive collections of shells, or particular kinds of dolls or stuffed toys, might be another sign.

Attwood notes that these differences in RRBIs between autistic females and males may be due in part to societal expectations and gender stereotypes. Autistic females may be more likely to be encouraged to engage in those activities stereotypically deemed socially acceptable for girls, while autistic males may be encouraged to engage in activities that are traditionally considered 'masculine'. Additionally, boys are not *dis*couraged from fascination with less socially acceptable items such as guns or weapons or war games. But there is, of course, no evidence that boys are encouraged to like weather patterns or the names of all the American presidents or to be obsessed with the number five. So perhaps the girls' 'nicer' obsessions reflect an additional, more general, factor at play – an element of the people-pleasing, ladylikeness mentioned in the context of internalizing behaviour. Be like other people and don't draw attention to yourself.

SENSORY PROCESSING AND FEMALE AUTISM

The inclusion of unusual sensory experiences in the official diagnosis of autism in 2013 has added another twist to the tale. As many as 90 per cent of autistic people report some kind of sensory sensitivities, so it is somewhat surprising that this was only included as a significant diagnostic sign in the latest version of DSM.[40] It now appears in the RRBI category as 'Hyper- or hyporeactivity to sensory input or unusual interests in sensory aspects of the environment (e.g., apparent indifference to pain/temperature, adverse response to specific sounds or textures, excessive smelling or touching of objects, visual fascination with lights or movement)'. There is increasing evidence that unusual sensory experiences are more common in females.

Imagine what your world might be like if your senses were tuned in an exquisitely different way. If your daily life was filled with sounds that were too loud, or lights that were too bright, smells too overpowering, clothes too scratchy, or tastes too powerful. Or, conversely, if your senses were tuned down too far, and you didn't react to sudden noises or the sound of your name. Or you were driven to unusual sensory-seeking behaviour: obsessions with certain textures, especially soft fabrics, or even licking or smelling surfaces or people (unfortunately not very acceptable in most social circles).

For example, here is one recollection from a woman called Jayne:

> When I was little, I loved to stroke soft things – rugs, dogs, peoples' clothes. If I saw something soft I just wanted to stroke it, I had to stroke it. It was alright at home but I did it anywhere we went. I think it was a time when fluffy jumpers were fashionable (angora, I think it was called). I went to the cinema with my mother and the girl in front had one of those jumpers on and I started to stroke it. She didn't like it and we had to move.

In light of the discussion above about 'underground' RRBIs in females, it is interesting to note that Jayne was quickly socialized out of this this particular habit: 'After that, my mother found me a piece of velvet that I could put in my pocket and stroke when I needed to, so nobody could see me'.

Fabric sensitivity is a common theme in the personal testimonies of autistic women. Temple Grandin was among the first to publicly offer a perspective on autism from the point of view of the autistic person. In her first autobiography, *Emergence: Labeled Autistic,* she writes that she would often refuse to wear certain clothing because of its texture, and that the feeling of scratchy fabric against her skin would cause her physical discomfort and distress. (She has since become an advocate for sensory-friendly design in clothing.) Parents of autistic girls have spoken to me about the piles of clothes that have had to be returned to shops because of scratchy labels or 'itchy' fabrics. One researcher, when I interviewed her about her autism, told me about her difficulties with her school uniform:

> I used to loathe the feeling of woollen tights on my skin. I could feel every individual fibre in the elastic, so when I sat down I felt like I was sitting on these really hard thin itchy bits of fabric and I could feel every individual bit of fibre and it was so uncomfortable it just made me cry.

It is becoming clear that that autistic females report significantly more sensory sensitivity than autistic males in all sensory modalities (i.e., auditory, visual, tactile, olfactory, and gustatory). A large-scale study in France showed that ASD children, both female and male, had higher scores than their typically developing peers on all the sensory scales.[41] There were no such differences between females and males within the neurotypical group, so the ASD differences were not just an expression of a general female-male difference.

Hypersensitive hearing is commonly reported as problematic for autistic people, and results in barriers to normal life, such as developing a dislike of going to restaurants because of the sounds of people chewing, or knives and forks clattering, or waiters taking orders. Christine McGuinness, a media celebrity and mother of three autistic children, was herself diagnosed as being autistic, having recognized so many of the diagnostic clues she heard from her children's clinicians. In the documentary *Unmasking My Autism*, she describes her discomfort at an award ceremony dinner where, as well as being anxious about a presentation she was due to make later in the evening, she was surrounded by an almost overwhelming medley of sights, smells, and sounds, with crowds of waiters milling about, the sounds of people eating, the smells of the elaborate dishes being served.[42]

Interestingly, in a study in 2021 looking at the characteristics of late-diagnosed autistic people, trying to find out if there were any key differences in how their autism had initially presented, the researchers found a much greater incidence of sensory differences among the late-diagnosed females than the males.[43] Remembering that sensory sensitivities as a defining characteristic of autism was only introduced in 2013, and noting that the females in this study were diagnosed an average of eight years later than the standard age of diagnosis, this is another example of diagnosticians looking at the wrong things – again, females weren't recognized because they had the 'wrong' symptoms.

STARTING TO ASK THE RIGHT QUESTIONS: WHAT IS IT LIKE TO BE AN AUTISTIC FEMALE?

The picture we have had of autism to date is broadly based on numerical outcomes of carefully scripted assessment protocols, tightly followed in brief, one-off orchestrated sessions. However, when you dig into the interviews with parents or carers more closely during such assessments, female differences become more evident. They, of course, are the people who would know the most about the everyday, real-life experiences of living with girls who may or may not be on the spectrum. And, it turns out, there can be quite a mismatch between the picture they draw of life with their autistic daughters and the output from assessment algorithms.

One mark of progress towards an understanding of the nature of autism in females is the emergence of assessments specifically designed to explore such differences. In 2011, psychiatric researchers Svenny Kopp and Christopher Gillberg were developing an add-on to an existing autism screening questionnaire specifically aimed at better capturing an autism phenotype in girls.[44] They identified a list of eighteen specific types of behaviour that their discussions with parents had identified as more characteristic of autistic girls. This covered patterns of behaviour such as copying or imitating other people's behaviour, avoiding demands, interacting mainly with younger children, episodes of eating problems, as well as 'extreme interest in pop/rock bands, soap operas or catastrophes involving large numbers of people'.

Similarly, as part of their campaign for better recognition of autistic girls, Tony Attwood and colleagues devised a questionnaire specifically to identify gender-sensitive profiles of autism characteristics. Having reviewed the emerging story of differently different autism in females, they identified questions for the parents of autistic children concerning those atypical behaviours that best might best characterize daughters as opposed to sons.[45] The idea was that these questions could be asked of the parents of both girls and boys, who would then indicate what was 'definitely not true' (score 1) to 'definitely true' (score 4). Those behaviours that best discriminated girls from boys ranged from certain kinds of sensory sensitivity ('Is s/he bothered by bright lights or certain kinds of lights [e.g., fluorescent light]?') to socialization issues ('Does s/he have many friends?', 'Is s/he shy in social situations?') as well as what could be called social identity issues ('Is s/he interested in looking feminine?/Is s/he interested in looking masculine?'). Once they tried out their questionnaire, they were able to group the answers under different headings in order to generate profiles that would differentiate autistic girls from boys.

'Sensory sensitivity' was one such heading, with parents of girls reporting a greater level of such difficulties. Another clue, then, that this could be an important part of females' autistic experience. There was also a greater level of 'social masking' and 'imitation' behaviour in girls, with parents noting their daughters copying other people's behaviour, or being markedly shy or silent in unfamiliar social situations. More on this later.

Another concern was to do with 'gendered behaviour'. This appears to be linked to gendered expectations of how girls or boys 'should' behave, with parents seemingly expressing greater concern if daughters rather than sons did not match up to the standard stereotypes. This fits in with the gendered socialization pressures we talked about earlier, where the pressures to conform are greater for girls and more attention is paid to violations of such expectations. I have also seen this strongly with my own work on the powerful role of gendered expectations in the socialization of girls – the very existence of a psychometric test called the Tomboy Index displays what a firm view the world has on what is 'appropriate' 'feminine' behaviour.[46] We will come across issues of gender identity and gender-incongruent behaviour later on, when we look at autism and adolescence.

The UK's Will Mandy and other key researchers in the world of female autism have had the inspired idea of harnessing a standard autism observational assessment schedule and revisiting the data from these assessments using a Gendered Autism Behavioural Scale (GABS) instead, or, in other words, a female spotlight![47] Drawing on a wide range of sources, including research findings and clinical reports as well as autistic autobiographies, the team drew up a coding system that identified four major categories of behaviour that, on average, picked out differences from what they called traditional autism phenotypes (which we might call the default male autism phenotype!).

The 'social adaptation' category covered evidence of individuals trying to mask typical autistic behaviour, such as stimming. It likewise covered conscious compensation for social difficulties – for example, individuals forcing themselves to make and maintain eye contact. 'Social relationships' focussed on friendships, the kind of friends they had (if any), and the extent to which they enjoyed social activities and interacting with others. 'Managing emotions' looked for evidence of both internalizing difficulties (being anxious or depressed) and externalizing, such as hyperactivity or aggression, but also looked specifically at responses to social acceptance or rejection – effectively how affected they were by such events. 'Interests and hobbies' tapped into RRBI-type information, asking about special interests or unusual preoccupations. Additionally, the researchers considered whether the interests were more social in nature (involving people or animals) or non-social (object-oriented interests in mechanism or machinery, or taxonomies such as timetables or weather patterns).

Trained coders then watched video recordings of standard ADOS assessments of groups of autistic males and autistic females and used the GABS framework to rate the occurrence of any of the behaviours covered by the four categories. It quickly became clear that GABS was picking up behaviours that were not captured by ADOS scoring. Females had higher overall scores on the GABS measures, with significant differences related to the emotional impact of acceptance or rejection, as well as higher levels of internalizing problems. This demonstrated that the traditional, male-oriented tests were missing key aspects of behaviour that are more common among females on the spectrum, and secondly, that there is a way of capturing these different differences. But only, of course, if you are looking for them!

From something of a standing start, we are beginning to get a clearer picture of autism's missing girls. One consistent variation from the traditional (male) autism phenotype is linked to the very core of autism itself – the notion that it is a problem with being social. The initial 'less than' approach to autism in females almost universally reports that social behaviour is less impaired in females. They appear to make more effort at making friends (although they do appear to struggle with maintaining such friendships). And the GABS study demonstrated that girls were more likely to be upset by social rejection, somewhat at odds with the notion that autism is associated with a lack of interest in social relationships. As we know, a greater awareness of gendered social norms and expectations has been put forward as an explanation for the less challenging presentation of autism in girls. However, this might seem paradoxical – why should anyone who, allegedly intentionally, shuts themselves off from society want to toe the social line?

If we look at the types of activities that come under headings such as GABS' social adaptation and social relationships, we can see patterns that are somewhat counter-intuitive in people who are traditionally characterized as having little or no interest in being social, fitting in with other people, or having friends. We find consistent reports of imitation, which can manifest as what looks like 'scripted' copying of other people's actions in social situations, or of understanding what makes friendships work or of actively seeking out and enjoying social activities.

There is a particular category of behaviour that has attracted more and more attention in the world of female autism, and that is the notion of masking or camouflaging, of actively trying to disguise autistic traits or of finding ways to blend in with non-autistic peers. Have autistic females found a way of masking or hiding their social problems, of compensating for their difficulties, of – chameleon like – developing some kind of protective camouflage that allows them to blend in? How do they do this? Perhaps more significantly, *why* do they do this and what impact does it have?

CHAPTER 4

BEHIND THE MASK

THE ART OF CAMOUFLAGING

As long ago as the 1980s, Lorna Wing suggested that the low numbers of women with an autism diagnosis might be because they had devised an elaborate form of camouflaging, an array of strategies and techniques that allowed them to not be noticed.[1] They had learned to 'hide in plain sight', rather like one of those moths that look like a piece of bark on a tree trunk. They had created a whole range of masks to hide behind, disguising their true identity or real responses to the outside world – anything as long as no one spotted that they were different or 'weird'. The aim of these strategies was to hide their true selves from others – their teachers, their peers, their friends, even their families – forever fearful of being found out.

Little attention was paid to pursuing this notion until the early years of this century, about thirty years after Wing's early suggestion. The main impetus came not from the clinical world or from research, but from the personal testimonies of autistic individuals, many of them late-diagnosed women, where camouflaging, or masking, or desperate attempts to blend in, were recurrent themes. They described their awareness of being different and of their urgent wish to hide this. They would detail how they painstakingly formulated social scripts – mimicking behaviour, copying verbal phrases or facial expressions, practising conversations – to avoid being 'othered' and excluded from society. They would almost obsessively prepare for dealing with the kind of everyday social situations most of us would automatically take in our stride. They referred to 'putting on my best normal' or 'hiding in plain sight', describing how much of their lives seemed to have been spent pretending to be the same as everyone else.[2]

One of the late-diagnosed autistic women I interviewed for this book described her experiences growing up as being like an undercover agent:

> I remember watching one of those war movies with my dad, where they were training spies to be dropped behind enemy lines. And they had to go undercover, and pretend to be a native of the country they were being dropped in. They could speak the language (which was why they had been picked) but they had to learn to behave exactly as if they were really Belgian or French or whatever it was. And they had days and days of training, where they had to read up about all about the country they were going to and the habits of the people and their quirky ways of behaving and talking. And they had to role-play and watch old films and newsreels really, really carefully and copy everything

exactly. And the trainers would set traps and try and catch them out. And they would only let them go and be spies when they had passed all these tests.

And there was one guy, an American, who had been perfect in training, and he was doing really well when he was dropped and had managed to meet up with the Resistance. But one day, he was sitting in a café, and these German soldiers came in. And the spy – the American – cut his food up with his knife and fork, and then he put his knife down and started to eat just with his fork. And only Americans did that so the Germans knew he was a spy and he was arrested.

And I realized my whole life till I was diagnosed was just like that, except I was going undercover without all the training and manuals and practice runs or newsreels to watch. I made up my own roles, writing little scripts for how to behave and not get caught, and I used to practice them in my bedroom in front of the mirror. And I'd go out and try to blend in and all the time I was panicking that the other girls would spot me – that I would forget and start eating with just a fork! And they wouldn't arrest me but they wouldn't let me join in any more and I would be on my own again . . . So I'd start every day terrified of what traps I might fall into, and go through the whole day on high alert.

This pattern of lifelong masking or camouflaging in order to belong to a group, or to avoid being spotted as different from other people, went unnoticed for a long time in the autism story. Indeed, if you think about it, it actually seems very much at odds with the traditional picture of autism, of individuals who appear somehow detached from the normal demands of social behaviour, indifferent to contact with other people. Aren't autistic people supposed to display little or no interest in adjusting their behaviour to ensure they fit in (or even any insight into the fact that they weren't)? A dawning awareness of this apparently paradoxical behaviour, in a group allegedly unlikely to be on the spectrum, means that the study of camouflaging behaviour has only recently emerged in the autism story.

WHAT IS CAMOUFLAGING? UNMASKING THE MASKING

The term 'camouflage' was first used in autism research writing in 2002, but it has really only been since about 2016 or 2017 that a steady stream of research publications devoted to discussions of autism and camouflaging has emerged.[3] Thanks to the efforts of psychologists such as Sarah Bargiela, Hannah Belcher, Helen Ellis, Francesca Happé, Laura Hull, Meng-Chuan Lai, Will Mandy, Victoria Milner, Elizabeth Pellicano, Felicity Sedgewick, and others we are starting to get a handle on the 'what' and the 'how' of this hidden aspect of autism.[4] As well as carefully constructing a rigorous research framework to guide their explorations, they have also pioneered the direct involvement of the autism community in their research. This involves not just tapping into the rich seam of personal testimonies that uncovered this previously unknown pattern of behaviour, but also consulting with autistic individuals on the construction of questionnaires and the interpretation of their findings.

The resulting investigations have revealed just how complex this pattern of behaviour can be. For example, masking is not the same as camouflaging. In their book, *Autism and Masking*, Felicity Sedgewick, Laura Hull, and Helen Ellis explain:

> Camouflaging is very much about hiding in the background and not being noticed, shying away for the spotlight and 'blending in' with the scenery. Not speaking up, not standing out, not being called upon, not being different. Masking is what takes place when camouflaging isn't possible and instead the survival strategy is about not being recognised as 'different' or 'struggling' and hiding true emotions and responses.[5]

The camouflager, then, might come across as extremely shy or quiet, never putting themselves forward, the girl in the corner, quietly tucking herself away from view. The masquerader, on the other hand, might come across as an extravert, or the class clown, or the performer, as illustrated in this personal account by Katy Wells in her book, *The Painted Clown*:

> I had been the geek, the book lover, the dancer, the academic, the sports fanatic, the food guru, the makeup expert. I had been whoever I needed to be. Whichever role I had played, had depended on who I had been with. My personas changed so readily. My survival had depended on my ability to adapt, to perform . . . to mask.

Other researchers have proposed a 'compensation hypothesis' linked to attempts to appear neurotypical, or 'pass as non-autistic' (sometimes referred to as PAN – you can tell when a concept is becoming more firmly embedded in academic research when it is awarded an acronym!).[6] They have described masking as something of a passive strategy 'just' attempting to hide the fact that you are not neurotypical – although *The Painted Clown* draws a picture of a rather exhausting creative energy at odds with this alleged passivity.

Compensation, on the other hand, is described as much more strategic.[7] The aim of compensation is not just to hide or blend in, but to generate 'as if' tactics that actually make you behave as if you were, indeed, neurotypical. So-called 'shallow' compensation includes the idea of identifying and following social rules, such as the appropriate length of eye contact, or generating specific scripts, such as how to show interest in other people's conversation by repeating phrases back to them, or by mirroring their body language. This is like the standard picture of camouflaging that emerges from autistic, lived experience testimonies, of how it involves harnessing powers of observation and imitation: *If I stand like the popular girl, and throw my head back when I laugh in the same way that she does, then I will be accepted and fit in like she does.* As one of the autistic teenagers I interviewed rather ruefully admitted, 'I'm hoping that if I walk like a neurotypical, and quack [sic] like a neurotypical, then maybe they'll think I am a neurotypical'.

'Deep' compensation concerns the notion that the social difficulties autistic individuals have are linked to their poor 'mind-reading' abilities, their lack of an automatic system of understanding other people, what those other people might be feeling or thinking, and how this might affect their behaviour. Deep compensation is an attempt to overcome such difficulties by trying to extract the 'principles' of social understanding, such as finding out how to interpret emotional expressions, how to pay attention to social cues, how to 'read the room'.

One of my adult female interviewees, who had recently experienced an unsatisfactory bout of social skills training entitled 'How to Read a Room', let loose an expletive-ridden rant at finding herself in a workshop where, having endured a round of less than helpful explanations of the difference between a genuine smile and a 'social' smile, she then found herself being told that the secret of social success was following the 7-38-55 rule: 7 per cent of social communication relies on the spoken word; 38 per cent comes from tone of voice; and 55 per cent from body language:

> Why can't it be 100 per cent the spoken word? Why can't people fucking say what they mean? How do I keep track of how long I've maintained eye contact at the same fucking time as listening to their 'tone of voice' – what does that even mean? – or checking to see if they are facing me full on or half turned away, and remembering which of those is a good thing or which a fucking bad thing?

HOW CAN YOU MEASURE CAMOUFLAGING?

By definition, successful camouflaging should be difficult to measure. Early research into camouflaging was almost entirely based on self-report, on camouflagers themselves describing when and how they behaved in particular ways, or responding to sets of questions. As we have seen, tremendous insights can be gained from such testimonies, although they naturally will involve self-selected, articulate adults. But there are important stories that are less accessible. Do children camouflage? If so, how young do they start? Autistic camouflagers almost invariably report that it was a strategy that they seemed to have always employed. Hannah Belcher, an autistic researcher who has written and spoken widely on her own experiences of being autistic, as well as researching the condition, describes her recognition of this pattern of behaviour:

> I realised I had been camouflaging my whole life. I'd been trying to mask my autistic traits and fit in with all the non-autistic people around me, desperate to always be liked and to never draw attention to myself.[8]

Psychologists have been tackling the problem of disentangling lifelong camouflaging practices from those problems that are being hidden. Existing tests were focussed on autistic presentation – either as measured by directly observing behaviour or as gleaned from interviewing parents or carers or, with respect to adults, the person themselves. A good score on social-interpersonal skills could mean that someone does indeed have good (or at least adequate) social-interpersonal skills and the autism red flag can be lowered. Or it could mean you are confronted with someone who has managed to hide their lack of such skills. Someone might look as if they have good interpersonal skills, but a little more detailed probing could show that these are not the product of what to a neurotypical might be effortless socializing.

Remember that many diagnosticians might see a child only once, in quite a controlled and contained situation, employing fairly standardized scripts and scenarios. If the child follows acceptable rules of social behaviour – for example, returns a greeting in an appropriate way, gives their name when asked, makes eye contact, answers questions, follows instructions and so forth – then the autism diagnosis may seem inappropriate. It may only be on a second meeting when the child behaves in exactly the same way, uses the same phrases even if the questions are slightly different, that the examiner might start to suspect that some kind of invisible social script is being followed. Or the parents might report that the teachers said the child had lots of friends but that she never got invited to their houses or any parties. Or the teachers might say the child was 'shy' or 'reserved' or not a 'joiner-in'. Or got very anxious if an unusual social event was being planned – such as a coach trip to London – and repeatedly pestered the organizers with urgent questions about where they would sit, who they would be next to, and why they were going, etc.

One labour-intensive but fruitful way of spotting camouflaging is by detailed observation of behaviour in real-life situations. Early researchers reported that if you watched social interactions very carefully, it was possible to spot almost imperceptible deviations from what looked like normal social behaviour, and that these might flag up nearly invisible social failures and attempts to deal with them.[9] In-person observation was particularly useful with children who might not have reached the stage of being able to report or reflect on their social difficulties, unless they were so disruptive that it was evident to parents or carers or teachers. In one study, researchers watched groups of both autistic and typically developing girls and boys as they played in their school playground.[10] They wanted to see the extent to which the autistic children might try and blend in to what was called their 'social landscape'. One thing that stood out was that the ASD girls spent much time 'flitting': moving from group to group of their peers, or 'hovering' on the edge of groups, perhaps seeming to be part of an ongoing game such as swinging a jump-rope but, on closer observation, never being given a turn to jump. ASD boys, on the other hand, were often spotted wandering alone, excluded from the structured games more characteristic of boy play. The researchers noted this difference as more problematic for ASD girls, as a casual observer might not spot that they were often being overlooked or failing to fit in with the ever-changing girl groups: they looked 'as if' they were socializing but were really on the outside looking in. One adult autistic female commented:

> Anecdotally, this is exactly the point of this behavior. When I was unconsciously masking as a child, my goal was always to appear like I was fitting in, even if I often felt very isolated by the fact that I wasn't actually fitting

in. As long as a random person watching me from the outside thinks I'm normal, then that's a victory.

What do these girls pick up during this flitting and hovering? We know that very young typically developing children have finely tuned social radar and are picking up on the rules of social engagement from an early age. For neurotypicals, understanding such rules seems to be so automatic and effortless that it is difficult to spot how this has happened (remember Alice's experience of her neurotypical son's behaviour in his first day at nursery?). But perhaps if you do not have that 'gift' of being social, the hard work starts early and can become a deeply ingrained part of your childhood memories. Autistic reminiscences often refer back to early struggles, as was shared with me by an autistic female who wasn't diagnosed until well into her forties:

> When I was at primary school, I remember hanging about on the edge of groups of girls. I was always trying to work out what the rules of the games were so I could join in. And I think I thought that playing by the rules were what the game was really about. Sure you could win by not getting caught or by doing the right number of jumps over the skipping rope, but you had to do it in the RIGHT WAY. I worked out one game and joined in and kept winning because I thought that the game was just about winning but they told me I wasn't following the rules properly and they stopped me joining in. And when I just watched them I saw they had changed the rules. So after that I made really sure that I didn't ever win as that seemed to be the rule they had made up for me.

This awareness of doing the wrong thing, of not fitting in, seems to emerge early. In the brutal world of childhood, being different can provoke overt bullying or the more subtle exclusion and ostracism. You don't have to be called 'weirdo' on the playground too many times, or find your desk filled with notes that 'no one likes you', to work out that you don't fit in. In the early years, the elaborate strategies of camouflaging or masking or script writing will probably be an unconscious response to this awareness, but the 'flitting' and 'hovering' could be taken as early signs of the need for close observation and mimicry. Trying to find the secret of 'doing the right thing' by watching those who seem to do it effortlessly emerges as a very early survival strategy. This was confirmed by one of my interviewees:

> When I was a young child, I went through a phase where I was terrified of going first in any group activity (and would have meltdowns if I was asked to do so). In hindsight, I was terrified at the prospect of having to demonstrate a behavior without first being able to observe and copy an 'acceptable' model of that behavior.

I once sat with a ten-year-old autistic girl in her school's quiet room, where she had been sent after an uncharacteristic outburst in class. She was staring out of the window at a group of girls and initially refused to engage me in any kind of conversation. I joined her in the staring for a bit and then asked her to tell me who these girls were and why they were interesting. What followed was a lengthy deluge of detailed information about each of the girls – how one told good jokes that made everyone laugh, how one was the most popular with the teachers (although she wasn't altogether sure why), and how one always seemed to be first with the latest fad. A sad little anecdote revealed how she hoped to use this information. My Little Pony toys were the latest must-have and she had saved up her pocket money to get the latest one so she could 'buy' her way into the friendship group she had been studying. Unfortunately, she hadn't noticed that the latest essential in the My Little Pony world was clip-on wings, so when she proudly produced her acquisition in the playground, it was just sneered at. And there was then a flurry of sarcastic comments about her new toy, well within earshot, of course. I asked if she would call her peers friends and she said she wasn't sure. They were going to a different secondary school from her at the end of the term and she said she didn't think they would miss her. All in all, it was a rather unhappy testimony to the mismatch between the aims and the outcomes of camouflaging behaviour.

Observation and interview have proved a rich source of material about camouflaging behaviour, hugely valuable at the individual level. Additional evidence is being provided by tests that offer more structured measures. One way of spotting camouflaging has been to measure the 'internal' signs of autism – perhaps by using scores on an autistic trait questionnaire, such as the Autism Spectrum Quotient or measures of emotion recognition – and then compare these scores with those from ADOS and/or ADI.[11] If there is a mismatch, or discrepancy, between how well someone might appear to be functioning socially (a 'pass' on a standard measure of autism) and the internal measures of how autistic they really are (high scores on a trait measure such as poor recognition of emotional expressions, or poor RMET performance), then this is a powerful clue that some kind of masking or camouflaging is in play.

These discrepancy measures were among the earliest used in the emerging study of camouflaging. A UK-based study in 2017, arising from a major collaboration between key autism research centres, reported that, on average, autistic females had higher camouflaging scores than males.[12] There was some evidence of camouflaging behaviour in males as well, so it mustn't be assumed that the researchers had lit upon some uniquely female behaviour in the autistic population. At this early stage, it wasn't possible to explore any qualitative differences between female and male camouflaging, such as when or how often it was used, and whether it involved the kind of intensive people-watching and shape-shifting that was being reported in the personal testimonies from autistic females. But that was to come.

A hybrid observation-interview-questionnaire approach was taken by Laura Hull, Will Mandy, and colleagues at University College London, who included autistic camouflagers in the development of their Camouflaging Autistic Traits Questionnaire.[13] The questions to be asked were elicited by talking to autistic people about their camouflaging activities, what they did, when they did it, and (importantly) why they did it. The researchers identified twenty-five items that seemed to reliably capture typical camouflaging behaviour. These comprised self-assessment statements such as, 'I have developed a script to follow in social situations', and 'I repeat phrases that I have heard other people say in exactly the same way I first heard them'.

They found that they could group the reasons for carrying out these kinds of behaviours under three headings. First, there are compensatory behaviours, which involve finding ways to learn skills that are not automatic ('I learn how people use their bodies and faces to interact by watching television or films, or by reading fiction'). Second, there is masking, or hiding autistic characteristics, which involves disguising 'inappropriate' autistic behaviour such as atypical emotional responses or lack of them ('I practise my facial expressions and body language to make sure they look natural'). Lastly, there is assimilation, which involves attempting to blend in by following some kind of rehearsed script ('In social situations, I feel like I'm "performing" rather than being myself'). Just the generation of these kinds of measures gives a feel for how complex camouflaging behaviour is and, perhaps paradoxically, the powerful insights into the rules and scripts behind social behaviour shown by these autistic contributors.

In 2021, a survey of camouflaging measures reported on sixteen different types of assessment that had emerged since the first experimental study in 2017.[14] From a standing start, the research community has shown a strong focus on this aspect of autistic behaviour. And across all the differing studies using tests of camouflaging, the evidence is accumulating that camouflaging is much more common in autistic females. A key aspect to notice here is evidence of a strong motivation to appear social in order to fit in. This feature is not in accord with the observations of Kanner and Asperger, and many since, that autistic individuals were deliberately or 'essentially' withdrawn, intentionally alone and aloof, and appeared to lack any kind of wish to belong to any kind of social network. The evidence of this chameleon-like behaviour in women and girls suggests there is a large piece missing from the autism jigsaw.

WHY DO WE CAMOUFLAGE?

As well as the 'what' and the 'how' of camouflaging, a more important issue is 'why'. Phrases such as 'putting on my best normal', 'I'm hiding behind what I want people to see', and 'I want to fit in with normal people' identify the need to at least appear to be like everyone else as a key driver for camouflaging. We encountered the PAN concept earlier on. Reading autistic personal testimonies suggests that PAN could equally well stand for 'pass as normal'. Belonging and fitting in are recurrent themes in discussions of camouflaging.

More widely, belongingness is a key concept in understanding human social behaviour, particularly our tendency to seek contact with other people, to form groups, and to work or play together.[15] The secret of human success is related to how we organize ourselves into groups. We solve problems collaboratively. We have found ways of understanding each other and working out the most successful kinds of social 'glue' that will keep groups together. At a personal or local level these could be friendship groups or peer groups or work-based teams.

Social psychologists have reported that the need to belong appears to be as powerful a motivational drive as basic survival instincts such as feeding or fight or flight. The term 'belongingness' has been coined to capture this need, of individuals craving to feel a sense of connectedness with other people.[15] There are powerfully negative effects if individuals are deprived of that sense of connection, if they are rejected or ostracized by the in-group to which they yearn to belong. These effects can be measured in plummeting levels of self-esteem, linked to social withdrawal and depression, even self-harm.

The autistic camouflaging drive to pass as normal, to develop a normal 'mask', could be a reflection of the need *not* to be rejected by other people, *not* to fail the team membership test, to be accepted as 'one of the girls'. Trying (and, sadly, failing) to understand the rules of how to make this happen is neatly summed up by one of my interviewees, fourteen-year-old Rachel, newly diagnosed as autistic, reflecting on her time at primary school:

> There was a group of cool girls that everyone wanted to join. I watched them a lot. I saw how close they stood

> to each other and how they all kind of circled round the leader and all laughed when she told a joke – you had to throw your head back in a particular way. And I listened to how she spoke and saw that she spoke differently to different girls. So I practiced all of this – really, in front of a mirror – and did what they did and tried to join in. But it didn't work and she got one of the other girls to come and tell me that no one liked me and that I was weird and to stop hanging around with them. . . . I think it's a bit like deaf people can't understand what sound is. They can see all the things like lips moving or people's heads turning in the same direction but they don't get that there's some kind of invisible something going from one person to another.

Linked to this need to belong is a wish to avoid the stigma of being 'not normal'. An online survey in 2022, looking at camouflaging behaviour and stigma consciousness, rated agreement or disagreement with statements such as, 'People knowing I am autistic does not influence how they act towards me'.[17] The survey demonstrated a clear relationship between stigma and camouflaging – the stronger your consciousness of stigma associated with autism, the more likely you were to display camouflaging behaviour. Camouflaging was described as a response to being 'othered' and feeling pressured to conform to non-autistic social conventions (and to avoid bullying and harassment).

In the neurotypical world, straightforward conformity, or aiming to just blend in, is akin to this. In the last chapter we looked at how the particular pressures of gendered socialization could powerfully shape patterns of behaviour in females. If there is a greater emphasis on girls, compared with boys, being socially compliant people-pleasers, it could translate into greater or more frequent efforts to camouflage atypical characteristics that might mark you as different. We noted in the last chapter that there was evidence that autistic females were more likely to find ways of suppressing or hiding stimming activities, which is another version of their masking and camouflaging behaviours.

Ironically, it has been suggested that the very notion of disguise might have negative consequences for camouflagers and perhaps even add to the stigma of being autistic. Wenn Lawson, a psychologist who is both autistic and transgender, has long focussed on issues for autistic females. He has noted that terms such as 'camouflaging' and 'masking' carry rather negative connotations of deceitfulness, or the need to hide something because it is somehow shameful. Instead he has suggested a rather unwieldy term, 'adaptive morphing', describing it as being like a chameleon.[18] Lawson suggests that the shape-shifting behaviour of autistic individuals is actually an instinctive, protective response to the perceived or actual harm that comes from being socially rejected or excluded. Indeed, the term 'survival response' is often applied by camouflagers (or adaptive morphers) when asked to sum up why they do it. They want to avoid the pain of social rejection. They want to escape the shame of being stigmatized as mentally ill or being 'othered' as weird or different.

DOESN'T EVERYBODY CAMOUFLAGE?

One issue that is often raised is whether or not camouflaging is somehow special to autistic women. As it has been suggested that camouflaging is a reason for the low levels of autism diagnosis in women, we need to identify if it is somehow distinct for this group, either in quality or quantity, or even in motivation.

The notion of camouflaging in neurotypical populations relates to what the social psychologist Erving Goffman called 'impression management'.[19] Impression management refers to the techniques and strategies employed to construct favourable impressions during social interactions. A key aim is to align your 'performance' with social norms and expectations, especially by the use of nonverbal cues such as facial expressions and gestures. These techniques seem to match some of those reportedly used by autistic camouflagers. But once you investigate when and where and how often neurotypicals behave in this way, it becomes clear that impression management is both quantitatively and qualitatively different from autistic camouflaging.[20]

Impression management is generally used in quite specific situations, such as job interviews or on first dates. More recently, clear evidence of impression management (and manipulation) has become pervasive on social media platforms, with carefully curated profiles highlighting positive attributes and achievements. But here we see instances of choice and control, with circumstances carefully selected. This behaviour is very unlike the intense and pervasive quality of autistic camouflaging, a process that seems near-permanently 'on' whenever the individual is in any kind of social situation. It has been reported that 70 per cent of autistic adults consistently camouflage, so for the majority it is definitely not a situation-specific, one-off, occasional pattern of behaviour.[21]

Don't autistic men camouflage? If that 70 per cent figure is accurate, then the answer would obviously be yes. But is their camouflaging different? There is a clear consensus from research findings that autistic females camouflage more often than autistic males, as measured both by self-report and structured and semi-structured questionnaire techniques.[22] Studies have reported that autistic males are more likely to report their camouflaging positively, describing it as easy and feeling it had achieved their aim of fitting in. Comments such as, 'a small sense of achievement and relief that it is over', or being pleased that the camouflaging has 'gone well' stand in stark contrast to reports of exhaustion and anxiety found in female personal testimonies.[23] Males are more likely to report that the aim of their camouflaging was to make friends and connect with others (which, again, is somewhat at odds with the traditional image of autism), whereas females were more likely to report that they were trying to avoid being ostracized or bullied, as well as trying to get by in educational or workplace settings. There is much more social anxiety associated with camouflaging in autistic females, which could reflect the greater pressure of gendered expectations at work.

So camouflaging is not unique to autism or to autistic females, but it figures much more frequently in females' behavioural profile, and appears to be aligned much more with conforming to social expectations (fitting in) and avoiding negative social experiences (rejection and ostracism, loneliness).

THE COSTS OF CAMOUFLAGING

You might think that an ability to hide social difficulties could be thought of as an autism superpower – an essential tool of a successful autistic undercover agent in a world of neurotypicals. The glimpses into the painstaking social detective work behind camouflaging or masking, the production of elaborate social scripts, the exhaustive rehearsals, and the hugely insightful self-reflection that the personal testimonies of autistic females have provided should earn a spark of admiration, at the least, for these camouflaging Chameleons. But there is a dark side to what on the surface might seem like effective adaptive behaviour.[24] Although the 'performance' might be sufficiently successful that the females' autism isn't spotted, the delivery of the performance turns out to be exhausting and dispiriting. This is a very common theme among women on the spectrum, describing the gruelling process of continuously monitoring and copying the social interactions that appear instinctive to their 'typical' peers, always on high alert in case they are 'caught'. Such experiences have been captured in the newer, interview-based research papers now providing a rich source of personal testimonies about what it is like to spend nearly all of your days 'pretending to be normal' or 'looking good but feeling bad'.[25] Women report being exhausted by the ongoing effort of monitoring how other people behave so they can formulate their own personal 'how-to' guides. They grow tired of constantly practising the mini-scripts they have generated so they can put on the right 'show', and of living in a chronic state of anxiety that they will be found out.

Autistic women's first-person accounts of the costs of camouflaging often report that, once they are alone, they may collapse in a heap, too tired to do anything. Young girls with autism, having held it together for the whole school day, often experience a post-school 'meltdown', turning into a 'snarling tiger cub' at the end of the day, giving way to tantrums, anger, and anxiety. When I talked to Becky, diagnosed as autistic at the age of six, she reflected on how she could be the 'good girl' at school but lost it once she got home:

> When I was in school, I would often have meltdowns after I got home. I would be able to hold it together during the day, but as soon as I got home, I would feel overwhelmed and exhausted. It was like I had been holding my breath all day and finally let it out. I would cry, scream, and sometimes hit myself. It was scary for my parents to see, and they didn't always know how to help me.

Such personal testimonies are borne out in research, which links camouflaging with mental health problems such as anxiety and depression. A survey in 2021 reviewed twenty-nine studies of camouflaging, including both self-report and the more objective discrepancy measures mentioned above, where there is a mismatch between the 'levels' of autism as measured by standardized tests (such as skills in emotion recognition) and observed performance.[26] The researchers confirmed that 'compared to autistic males, autistic females reported camouflaging across more situations, more frequently and for more of the time'. They also confirmed a relationship between camouflaging and poor mental health, including increased social anxiety, depressive symptoms, burnout, and suicidal thoughts.

Many studies have reported on the negative relationship between camouflaging and psychological well-being. A process that should help you pass as normal or escape bullying and loneliness comes at a price. Given the consistent reports on the higher levels of camouflaging in autistic women, we should not be surprised to find surveys reporting that about 20 per cent of autistic women are hospitalized for a psychiatric condition by age twenty-five, a figure more than five times higher than for women without autism and more than twice that of autistic men.[27] When we add into the mix that camouflaging behaviour is strongly linked to the kind of internalizing behaviour that is characteristic of those mental health problems, such as anxiety and depression, that are more common in females, we can really get a feel for the high price autistic women are paying for 'putting on their best normal'.

There is clearly a strong force driving autistic women to camouflage. Camouflaging is not a sign of autism in itself, but it is evidence of a powerful motivation to disguise social difficulties, or to compensate for the lack of social know-how that seems to come automatically to the neurotypical population. The motivation is so powerful that camouflaging will continue in the face of physical exhaustion and severe mental health challenges.

So far in the book, we have been trying to find out why and how females on the spectrum have largely been missed in the autism story, and to see if we can fill in the details of what autism in this neglected group might look like. We have seen that the image of a 'paler' version of male autism, or of a group whose social training has just masked or muffled the more challenging aspects of autism, does not stand up to closer scrutiny.

The camouflaging story presents a pattern of behaviour completely at odds with the traditional image of social withdrawal and isolation. It indicates the presence of a highly complex sleuthing system that can code and mimic the rules of social engagement, construct social scripts, and learn how to play elaborate social roles. Moreover, it indicates the presence of a powerful social motivation that will drive the application of such skills even at the cost of mental and physical health. The human need to be social is certainly present in this group of individuals, playing out even more powerfully than in their neurotypical peers.

The next part of the story takes us into my world, the world of the brain. Autism is a brain-based problem, although currently only identifiable by patterns of behaviour. One area of focus in the search for autism in the brain has, understandably, been the social brain, the neural underpinnings of typical and atypical social behaviour. We have seen that camouflaging is a highly complex type of social behaviour, more common, on average, in autistic females. So perhaps a closer look at what brain researchers have to say about autism in the brain might offer some more clues about autism in women.

PART II

THE BRAINS BEHIND IT ALL

CHAPTER 5

THE AUTISTIC BRAIN

TO BEGIN AT THE BEGINNING

When I ask autistic people what question they would most like neuroscientists to answer, the most common response is simply 'How do autistic brains get to be autistic?' While the question itself is clear, answering it is a daunting task. Perhaps the best place to start is by taking a step back and looking at the biological coding that shapes the brain's development: genetics. Where does autism come from?

From the outset of the awareness of autism, it was clear that it tended to run in families. Early clinical case notes included detailed reference to the behaviour of parents and close relatives, in particular those aspects of behaviour that might be dubbed unusual. When Kanner asked Donald Triplett's father to tell him a bit more about Donald, he received thirty-three closely typed, single-spaced pages, which Kanner noted as 'obsessive'.

Having one autistic child greatly increases the chances of having another. The idea that there was some heritable factor at play was established early on, but it was not really until the 1970s that it became a focus of autism research.[1] As is so often the case in the study of genetic investigations, the research focussed on twins. This is because twins would normally be exposed to the same sort of environmental factors, including parenting styles. If identical twins (sharing nearly 100 per cent of their genetic material) were more similar with respect to some kind of physical or mental characteristic than non-identical or fraternal twins (sharing 50 per cent on average), it would provide strong evidence that the characteristic was genetically determined.

The UK psychiatrist Michael Rutter set out to recruit as many sets of twins as possible, where either one or both had been diagnosed as autistic. With the help of his co-worker Susan Folstein, an American physician, he tracked down twenty-one pairs of same-sex twins with confirmed autism diagnoses.[2] Eleven were identical twins and ten were fraternal. Of the identical twins, four pairs were both identified as autistic. There were no such pairings in the non-identical group. Rutter followed up this work twenty years later. With a much larger sample of twins, he found a 60 per cent occurrence of autism in both twins among the identical twin pairs, as compared to (again) 0 per cent in the non-identical twins. When he and his team looked in more detail at specific symptoms associated with autism, such as social and language skills, they found even higher so-called concordance rates of 82 per cent in the identical twins. It was clear that genetic factors must have a major role to play in the causes of autism.

Studies have indicated that autism is one of the most heritable of all mental health conditions, with heritability estimates ranging from 50 to 90 per cent. This means that, if you are looking at variability in an autistic population, a lot of the variation can be attributed to genetic factors. It's important to realize that heritability refers to how much of any particular characteristic – be it autism or eye colour – seems to be determined by genetic factors. This isn't the same as saying that the brother or sister of an autistic child has a 50 to 90 per cent probability of being autistic, although the likelihood could be increased as they may share some of the relevant genes. This is why some autism researchers might also recruit the siblings of autistic children, to see what brain or behavioural characteristics they might share.

Any characteristic that a geneticist studies is known as a phenotype. Effectively it concerns what a particular characteristic looks like, or how it presents to the outside world. Eye colour, for example, is one of the easiest phenotypes to study as there is pretty much universal agreement as to the difference between, say, brown eyes and blue eyes. Blood type is slightly trickier, as it involves a special test, but there is, again, universal agreement as to the difference between type A and type O. One of the main difficulties that genetic researchers in the autism field have is about the phenotype of autism. The matter brings us back to the question asked in the first chapter – what is autism? Or perhaps we should say, what does autism look like? We are not (as yet) looking at any agreed-upon physical characteristic – we are talking about different types of behaviour and the extent to which these might be viewed as atypical. How might you measure these to let the geneticists know what they are looking for?

If we remind ourselves of how clinicians arrive at a diagnosis of autism (which we already know is not what one might call an exact science), the problem immediately becomes obvious. To meet diagnostic criteria for ASD according to DSM-5, a child should have persistent deficits in each of three areas of social communication and interaction, which could include their conversation skills or understanding of relationships. The manual includes examples of these, which we're told are 'illustrative, not exhaustive'. The deficits have to be ranked on three different levels of severity. Then there are four kinds of restricted, repetitive patterns of behaviour (including insistence on sameness, obsessive and narrow interests, hyper- or hypo-sensitivity), of which the person must have at least two (but it could be any two, which, of course, instantly increases the amount of variability). Similarly, there are illustrative but not exhaustive examples. And again, these behaviours should be ranked on one of three levels of severity. You might like to ponder just how many different pictures of autistic behaviour might be produced by the above combinations. And this is without adding to this mix what we now know about how many different pictures of autistic behaviour have actually been *missed* by these elaborate criteria: i.e., the differing picture of autism in women and girls. The phrase we've come across before – 'If you've met one person with autism, you've met one person with autism' – brilliantly sums up the uniqueness of autistic people, but it also sums up the formidable task geneticists are faced with.[3]

Their frustrations are voiced by the cognitive neuroscientist Ralph-Axel Müller from San Diego State University:

> If there has been failure that has prevented the science of ASDs to generate mechanistic models of causation . . . , it is a failure to appreciate the inadequacy of a clinical label such as 'autism spectrum disorder' in the pursuit of neurobiological causes. From a developmental neurobiology perspective, the expectation that a consensus-based catalog of behavioral observations (as listed in the DSM-5) could tractably correspond to a small set of genetic causes or brain features is misguided.[4]

This is frustrated researcher-speak for 'If you think we can extract a simple biological explanation for autism from the jumble of shape-shifting definitions provided by decades of diagnostic wrangling, you've got another thing coming.'

Once we start to investigate brain structure or function in autism, the problems are multiplied. There are 86 billion neurons in the typical human brain; structural connections between them are estimated at 100 trillion. Functional brain networks are indexed by measuring frequencies ranging from 0.5 Hz to over 100 Hz, divided into five different bands. There are twenty to twenty-five thousand protein coding genes in the human genome (and let's not even get into the many thousands of non-coding genes, which actually comprise 97 per cent of the human genome) and approximately three billion base pairs. Combine that with the hugely heterogenous and (if you are in Ralph-Axel Müller's camp) inadequately defined condition that is autism, and you might wonder where even to begin.

And if that wasn't enough, there is the 'you can never bake the same cake twice' issue in genetics. This helpful insight into the complexities of inheritance, from the geneticist Kevin Mitchell, introduces us to the mysteries of 'developmental variation'.[5] We're familiar with the picture of the two long strands of the DNA molecule that coil around each other to form what looks like a twisted ladder, the double helix, with each of the 'rungs' made up of pairs of the four key chemical bases – adenine (A), thymine (T), cytosine (C), and guanine (G). And we've probably seen many cartoon images showing how DNA reproduces, with the ladder-like structure unwinding and dividing neatly down the middle of its rungs, and each half-rung then picking up its missing pair, making two new DNA ladders. These images often leave the impression that the result of DNA division will be an exact replica of the original. Not so.

The human genome has three billion of these chemical bases to be replicated when DNA divides and there can be many 'spelling mistakes'. These mistakes can involve a single letter, an 'A' not being paired with a 'T', for example, or maybe a short 'run' of letters not picking up their usual pairs. Or a strand of DNA that gets deleted or relocated. The system has an inbuilt proofreading or error-correcting function, but mistakes still happen. So, after replication, the new DNA will be just that very tiny bit different, not usually enough on its own to make any physical difference unless it affects the function of a single key gene, as in the case of cystic fibrosis, for example. But if there are many such spelling mistakes, the outcome of these very slightly different ingredients could be a dramatically different cake. So genetic detective work mainly involves trawling through the genome and looking for spelling mistakes. As it turns out, many of the gene changes implicated in autism are such single-letter changes or copying mistakes, so there are many tiny little variations whose contribution to the end-product will be really hard to pin down. And when that end-product is as inadequately defined as autism and encompasses such a huge range of possible presentations, you might wonder why anyone would embark on such a Herculean task.

But autism researchers have persisted, greatly assisted in recent years by stunning advances in genetics research techniques, exponential leaps in computing power, the sequencing of the human genome, and the emergence of large-scale collaborative research consortia dedicated to unpicking the autism puzzle.

HOW DO WE LOOK FOR GENETIC FACTORS IN AUTISM?

If we look at as many people with autism as possible, ideally testing their close relatives as well, we might be able to see if any consistent pattern of genetic anomalies emerges. We will, of course, encounter the variability problem, but given the increasingly fine-grained detail that geneticists are able to extract from their data (and the enormously powerful machine-learning techniques now available), this problem is less daunting than it used to be. Some studies are monumental in scale. For example, one recent Danish study looked at data from almost the entire Danish population born between May 1, 1981, and December 31, 2005, among which the researchers identified over eighteen thousand autism cases.[6]

In addition, there are known developmental disorders where the genetic cause has been identified that present with patterns of atypical behaviour very similar to those of autism. These can offer clues as to how a particular genetic blueprint might be linked to the kind of behavioural anomalies that are also true of autism. One example is Rett syndrome, which, if you recall, was once bracketed with autism in an early DSM version. Some conditions exhibit both behavioural and brain-based characteristics closely similar to those of autism. One example is Phelan-McDermid syndrome, a rare genetic condition linked to the deletion of a particular gene, the SHANK3 gene, on chromosome 22.[7] This gene plays a crucial role in the development and functioning of nerve cell connections in the brain, which, as we shall see, appears to be a key problem in the autistic brain. Children with this condition show many of the same behavioural problems as autistic children – in fact, many would 'pass' the diagnostic threshold for autism if it had not already been determined that they had Phelan-McDermid syndrome.

Another way of looking for genetic influences in autism is to manipulate a genome and see what happens to the phenotype. Obviously, you could not do this in humans, so this is where animal models of autism come in. The aim is to produce 'symptoms' of autism in mice or rats or zebrafish (or even fruit flies) by 'knocking out' targeted genes and seeing what happens to their behaviour. Mice are popular candidate animals in genetic research because mice and humans share a significant portion of their genetic material, and many of the genes associated with autism in humans have counterparts in mice. The mouse brain also shares many structural and functional similarities with the human brain. Studying the effects of genetic modifications on the mouse brain can provide valuable information about how similar changes might affect the human brain. As mice have short reproductive cycles, researchers can study multiple generations relatively quickly.

What, you might ask, does an autistic mouse or even an autistic fruit fly look like? As they both have quite sophisticated patterns of social behaviour, we can see if these are disrupted by genetic changes. For example, if you knock out the SHANK3 gene, mentioned previously, mice will exhibit several unusual behaviours reminiscent of autism, including differences in social interaction, with reductions in normal 'getting to know you' activities such as nose-to-nose sniffing or grooming.[8] In fruit flies, researchers can measure 'social-space behaviour'. How close do flies get together? How often do they follow or touch each other? They can then investigate how these behaviours are disrupted by manipulating genes.

The advantage of such studies is that they can directly test the causal effects of gene alterations. The disadvantage is, of course, that they are unlikely to capture the true essence of being autistic. However, they may provide another piece of the jigsaw.

WHAT HAVE WE FOUND?

SHANK3; SYNGAP1; NRXN1; CNTNAP2; CHD8; PTEN; TSC1; TSC2; MECP2; FMR1; NLGN3; NLGN4X; DYRK1A;

ADNP; GRIN2B; SCN2A; ANK2; FOXP1; NR2F1; PCDH10; SHANK2; SHANK1; AFF2 (FMR2); NR3C2; PTCHD1; MET; RELN; OXTR; GABRB3; GABRA4; TBR1; JAKMIP1; UBE3A; KCDT13; MAP3; KCNN2; KMT2C; PTBP2; MTHFR; SLC25A12; VDR.[9]

In case you think I have fallen asleep face down on my computer keyboard, I should let you know that these are just some of the hundreds of genes that, to date, have been implicated in autism. The current confirmed count is over a thousand, at least one for every chromosome, and it is predicted there will be more to come. There is, of course, no such thing as a single autism gene, which is unsurprising given the many variables we talked about previously. But common factors are, painstakingly, being identified.

For example, we've seen that one gene, SHANK3, is powerfully implicated in both social behaviour and in building brain networks, especially at the synapses, the connections between nerve cells. This provides a clue that brain researchers might like to focus on pathways in the brain. Other genes that have been identified, such as CNTNAP2 and RELN, are also closely involved in proteins that are involved in nerve cell development and, in particular, the connections between nerves.[10]

The Simons Foundation, which monitors and supports autism research, now runs an astonishing 'live' database into which any gene associated with autism susceptibility is entered and scored for the strength of the evidence linking it to the development of autism. You can 'click' on each chromosome to find out what genes have been implicated and what those genes are responsible for.[11] So although there is, as yet, no answer to the 'where does autism come from?' question, it is certainly not for want of trying.

THE FEMALE PROTECTIVE EFFECT?

One particular focus in early genetics research has been the alleged 'female protective effect'.[12] What was behind the widely accepted 'fact' of a 4:1 male-to-female ratio in autism? One line of enquiry was the possibility that female biology offered some kind of protection, some kind of buffer against autism. This could be hormones or something that determined their brain wiring was less likely to go awry. Of course, as this book has shown, the lack of women diagnosed with autism has often more to do with failures in how autism is diagnosed and understood, as opposed to a reflection of the real prevalence of autism in women. But, let's not throw the baby out with the bath-water. If there is any possibility that there are some sex-related factors at work in who is or isn't autistic, then we must pursue them.

Biological females have two X chromosomes, and males have only one. Normally, only one of a female's X chromosomes is activated during early embryonic development, with the genes on the inactivated chromosome effectively silenced. This means that if there are any mutations (for good or ill) on the silenced chromosome, they won't be expressed in the phenotype, and the female won't display the effect of the mutation (although she can be a carrier). As boys only have one X chromosome, they don't have this possible 'escape' route. So an obvious focus for any female protective effect in autism would be to look at genes on the X chromosome.[13]

There are genes on the X chromosome that are known to play crucial roles in brain development and nerve cell function. NLGN3 is one of the genes responsible for producing neuroligins, proteins that function in the synapses. Any kind of problem here could be linked to the efficiency of key networks in the brain. Given that this is a gene found on the X chromosome, there has been some speculation as to its role in the apparent sex bias in autism.[14] But it has also been implicated in the genotypes of other developmental disorders, so it is not autism specific.

There is another gene located on the X chromosome whose effects have been strongly linked to autism. This is the FMRI gene. Mutations in this gene cause so-called 'Fragile X syndrome', another neurodevelopmental disorder linked to autism-like behavioural challenges.[15] This gene normally produces a protein that is needed for brain development, particularly for laying down neural circuits. About 30 per cent of children with Fragile X syndrome also meet the clinical criteria for autism, and often show the same kind of social communication difficulties, repetitive behaviours, and sensory sensitivities. Both males and females can have Fragile X syndrome, but it tends to be more common and more severe in males. So, it is certainly worth tracking abnormalities in the FMRI gene in autistic individuals.

If there is a female protective effect, we have not yet discovered the smoking gun on the X chromosome. But another way of looking at this issue is to ask a more indirect question. If it is (apparently) harder for females to 'get' autism, is there any evidence that females who have been diagnosed as autistic have had to have collected a greater number of genetic anomalies before their autism-protective biology is breeched?[16]

The hypothesis that those rare females who were diagnosed with autism might display a greater genetic 'hit' first arose in the 1980s when it was noted that autistic girls had, on average, more autistic relatives than did autistic boys. To geneticists, this suggested a greater number of 'available' autism-related gene mutations, a richer atypical gene pool. Additionally, siblings of autistic girls had a higher risk (44 per cent) of being autistic than those with autistic brothers (30 per cent) – again, a clue that such families had a more prolific autism gene pool. Similarly, in non-identical twin pairs, the male of a twin pair was much more likely to be autistic if his sister was autistic than if his brother was. All these findings suggest that there are a higher number of genetic anomalies associated with being an autistic girl, reflected in the wider range of autism-type differences in her family.

Several studies using a range of different genetic exploration techniques have explored the occurrence of different mutations in the genomes of male and female autistic participants. Their findings do strongly support the notion of much higher rates of genetic anomalies in autistic females – a 'higher mutation burden'. It seemed that females do indeed need to be hit harder before they present as autistic.

It is unlikely that we will ever map out a complete genetic blueprint for autism, although a focus on different aspects of the condition might prove fruitful. If I could dictate a genetic research focus, unsurprisingly, I would want the genes behind structural and functional pathways in the brain, particularly those linked to key aspects of autistic behaviour, to be explored. What do we know about genetic effects on pathways in the social brain, for instance? How soon do these genetic anomalies exert their effects on the autistic brain? To answer such questions, we need to start our investigations as early as possible in life.

THE FIRST ONE THOUSAND DAYS: PATHWAYS IN THE BRAIN

When we look at behavioural disorders that are present from birth and clearly affect typical development, we need to find ways of tracking when and where things go awry. This is especially so if, as with autism, the condition is not accompanied by any external physical signs that might serve as an early warning sign of unusual brain development, such as is the case with Down syndrome. The only way we can identify autism is by behaviours that generally don't become evident until the second year of life, and which may not result in a clinical diagnosis until a child is three years old or even, as we have seen, much later, especially in girls. Autistic differences and difficulties do not, as one researcher has observed, 'appear abruptly as with the flip of a switch'; they have always been there. So, during those first three years (or one thousand days) of life, there is something in the developing autistic brain that will be the precursor to all the downstream issues.[17] This is where we should start if we hope for full answers to the question of what makes autistics autistic.

The brain at birth is relatively under-wired; a brain scan in a newborn will mainly show up as areas of grey matter, marking the bodies of the nerve cells or neurons, already grouped into different brain structures. The stunning growth that occurs in baby brains from birth is almost entirely due to the laying down of neural pathways that occurs throughout childhood to adulthood, with something of a reboot occurring during adolescence. Axons, the long slender projections on nerve cells, will be reaching out for their predestined targets, growing multiple branching receiver sites or dendrites. There are some great YouTube videos that really bring this process to life![18] As axons develop they become wrapped in a fatty substance called myelin, which increases the speed at which electrical signals pass along the axon. Myelin shows up as white matter in brain scans, so tracking the increase in white matter reveals how efficiently (or not) a brain is being 'wired up'.

Early brain scanning studies mainly focussed on grey matter, assuming that the size of a structure might give a clue as to its effectiveness. As you might imagine, these kinds of 'size matters' arguments figured prominently in debates about 'male' and 'female' brains. But now the focus is much more on the connections within the brain, both structural and functional, so-called connectomics.[19] The ability of brain-imaging techniques to map connections in the brain, as well as just structures, can produce hugely detailed brain 'road maps' that tell us the size and strength of the white matter tracts, some comprising millions of axons. But we can also look at dynamic connections, the flow of information along the different pathways, rather like watching those speeded-up films of car headlights at night.

In the developing infant brain, many millions of synapses, the interconnection sites between nerve cells, will be formed, almost twice as many, in fact, as are found in the adult human brain once it has stopped growing – a vigorous pruning process occurs later in childhood and adolescence. Developmental disorders such as autism have often been linked with variations in the extent and the rate of early brain growth in both grey and white matter, and also with the slowdown and reversal of growth in late childhood and adolescence. As we shall see, some brains grow much more dramatically than others and show much less evidence of the pruning or tidying-up processes that occur at the end of a brain's developmental trajectory.

From the early days of studying autism there were clues about abnormal brain development. Kanner noted that five of the children he studied had large heads, and, much later, this became a focus of some of the initial brain studies of autism.[20] Championed by Eric Courchesne from the University of California, San Diego, head circumference was used as an indirect measure of brain size. There are many images of Courchesne and his colleagues earnestly slipping everyday tape measures around babies' heads and recording their measurements. Despite the rather phrenological overtones, it turned out that head size might be a useful early clue.

Courchesne's findings led him to suggest a pattern of dramatic early brain overgrowth in autistic children up until about four years of age, followed by abnormally slow or arrested growth. This would coincide with the age at which networks are being formed in the developing brain, with the autistic brain showing an over-enthusiastic 'road-building' programme between just about any and all brain structures. Courchesne suggested that the 'exuberant overgrowth' in the autistic brain could result in disruption or reduced efficiency, leading to the downstream behavioural problems characteristic of autism.

This was a clue that something was going awry early on in autistic brains, well before a diagnosis of autism might be triggered. But it was obviously only a very indirect and rather crude clue. How might the brain of a baby who went on to develop autism be different from the brain of one who didn't? When and where might the road building programme have gone wrong? The ideal solution would be to scan the brains of a large population of babies at regular intervals and then look back at those scans if any of them developed autism. In the early days of autism research this obviously wasn't practically (or financially) possible. This where the so-called 'high-risk' studies came in.[21] High-risk studies are research studies that focus on individuals who are at an increased risk of developing a particular condition due to certain predisposing factors, but who do not currently present with such a condition. These studies aim to identify early markers, understand the developmental trajectories, and explore the underlying mechanisms that might lead to the onset of the condition.

Given that heritability had been established as at least 50 per cent and maybe higher, it was clear that there was a much higher chance that any subsequent siblings of autistic children might themselves be autistic. In the general population, the occurrence of autism is nearly 2 per cent; in the siblings of autistic children, the risk rises to between 10 and 20 per cent. Knowing this is important for discussions with the families of autistic children. Additionally, it offers the research community a convenient pool of infants and children who may or may not go on to develop autism. It is in the months immediately after birth during which the typical or atypical development of many thousands of brain connections takes place, so investigating the brains of babies who may, or may not, go on to develop autism can be a hugely valuable source of clues.

Another advantage of high-risk studies is that they give us a better chance of separating early biologically determined characteristics from the potentially brain-changing consequences of living life as an autistic person. If the world is too loud or too bright or too smelly, it is hard to pay attention to the to and fro of everyday conversations, and you may fail to pick up key social clues. Or the world might not understand your differences, and you may be bullied or just ignored in later life. All these experiences can alter how brains develop, so researchers need to get to at-risk brains as soon as we can.

Once it became possible to use brain imaging in infants as a direct measure of brain development, evidence was revealed, in some autistic children at least, of enlarged brain surface area and volume, consistent with Courchesne's suggestion of overgrowth.[22] The accelerated growth was shown in both grey and white matter, in particular in the white matter tracts that mark the pathways within and between different areas in the brain. Most baby autism studies have reported patterns of over-connectivity in the early years of autistic brain development, especially within developing local networks. This might present as heightened activity within sensory systems, for example, and could be the basis of the sensory difficulties that we know are so common in autism. In typically developing brains, the next stage would be establishing more long-distance connections, so there can be a richer and more co-ordinated response to incoming information. Animal models have shown that unusually high levels of localized connectivity can derail this next stage, and long-distance connections form more slowly and less effectively. There doesn't seem to be any fixed pattern as to which brain pathways are disrupted and when, just that it is a characteristic anomaly in those at-risk infants who subsequently are diagnosed as autistic. This could underlie the very mixed pattern of differences and difficulties within the autistic population.

You can measure how efficient developing networks are in infant brains by looking at the length and strength of the structural pathways. Consistent with atypical patterns of activity that have been measured, it is clear that the developing pathways in the brains of infants at risk for autism show much lower levels of efficiency.[23] In one longitudinal study, the researchers were able to compare the earlier measures of network efficiency in a group of twenty-four-month-old high-risk children who had themselves been diagnosed with autism. They showed that the lower the efficiency scores measured at six months and twelve months of age, the higher the autism symptom severity scores at twenty-four months.

In 2020, there was an exciting development in this quest. A team from King's College London, using specialist fMRI techniques, managed to measure patterns of connectivity in the brains of forty newborn infants, twenty of whom were at high risk of developing autism, having a first degree relative with autism, and twenty of whom were carefully matched controls, with no such family history.[24] The at-risk infants showed significantly higher levels of local connectivity within a wide range of brain areas, especially in sensory areas. There was no difference in long-range connectivity between the two groups, supporting the idea that the formation of more widespread networks comes later in the developmental journey of autistic brains. The researchers have speculated that this atypical brain connectivity measured at birth might serve as some kind of biomarker, identifying which brains might be more vulnerable to later, more extensive 'wiring' problems. The next stage of this work will involve exploring how these early brain differences might be reflected in later atypical cognitive and behavioural presentations consistent with an emerging picture of autism.

The story that these technologically advanced studies of tiny brains is telling is that, in autism, something goes awry very early on with the establishment of crucial brain connections, certainly from birth and quite possibly even from conception. This would fit in with the genetic evidence, which has shown that many of the candidate genes related to autism are responsible for ensuring accurate and effective nerve cell connections in the developing brain. There appears to be no distinguishing time or place at which things start to deviate from the norm (remember we are looking at over a thousand possible genetic culprits), which could account for the wide range of symptom patterns and levels of severity.

Studies of brains in autistic adults tell a somewhat similar story as those of infant and toddler brains. Some (but not all) adult brains show the same evidence of brain overgrowth into adulthood, linked to greater increases in the surface area of the brain's grey matter. So, in some cases, the early exuberant growth (and the associated problems) is not corrected in the adult brain by the kind of vigorous pruning and pathway selection that we see in non-autistic brains.

Early studies of brains in autistic adults focussed on specific structures, such as the amygdala, a key part of emotional control networks in the brain, but no consistent findings have emerged.[25] The most promising findings, as in the study of infant brains, have emerged from studying connections in the brain, the physical pathways but also the ebb and flow of information between them. If we really want to understand the relationship between our brains and our behaviour, typical or atypical, then we need to map the brain activation patterns associated with whatever behaviours we are interested in, where they come from and when, where they go to and when. We will return to this in the next chapter.

SEX DIFFERENCES IN THE AUTISTIC BRAIN

A key question for this book is whether or not any of these studies of autistic brains have come across any sex differences. And here, of course, we come up against the male spotlight problem again. It turns out that, unlike the eager 'hunt the sex difference' crusades over many years in the study of neurotypical brains, autism research has, until relatively recently, avoided the difficulties associated with studying two sexes by just studying the one.[26] We have already encountered the rather startling statistic, from a survey of twenty years of neuroimaging autism research published in 2021, that in a group of over 1,400 studies from this era, 30 per cent of them tested only males. Seventy-seven per cent of the remaining studies, even though females were included, didn't test for sex differences (almost invariably because so few females were included), or sex was controlled out of the analysis as a nuisance variable![27]

But the 'call to arms' led by Meng-Chuan Lai in 2015 does seem to have improved this state of affairs, with a steep rise in the number of publications highlighting sex differences in autistic brains.[28] Just over three hundred studies were published between the year 2000 and 2015. Between 2015 and 2024 this number rose to over 750. Has anything emerged?

The most consistent indication of potential sex differences refers to the 'big head, big brain' story. Firstly, increasing evidence shows the head size issue is relevant in only about 20 per cent of autistic boys.[29] And it appears that, where there is evidence of brain overgrowth, it is much stronger in young autistic boys and this difference is sustained until adulthood. It is more common for autistic girls to show similar trajectories of brain development to neurotypical girls early on, but then show less of the normal pruning-related decline during adolescence. In fact, the strongest emerging theme from the last ten years or so is that any sex differences could be age-related, and may only be evident in certain developmental time windows. So in the search for key structures that might underpin sex differences in autism, detailed follow-up studies across the lifespan will be needed.

As we know, the notion of the female protective effect in autism has been tested by looking at the number of genetic anomalies in girls diagnosed with autism as compared to boys. The findings suggested that girls did indeed 'need' a higher mutational hit rate before they passed the clinical threshold. Researchers wondered whether or not this might be reflected in a higher number of brain atypicalities in autistic girls as compared to boys.

One study looked at twin pairs where only one of the twins was autistic, to see if there were any differences between their brains.[30] There were five female pairs (two identical and three non-identical) and eleven male pairs (five identical and six non-identical). No differences were found between the autistic females and males with respect to the severity of their autistic symptoms. Comparing the brains of the female twin pairs, scan differences showed up in eleven different regions of the brain, with the autistic twin showing reductions in the volume of these regions. In the male twin pairs, there were differences in only two, slightly different, areas. So, echoing the genetic findings, girls could be carrying a greater number of brain differences than boys while outwardly displaying the same level of symptoms. Obviously, this was a very small-scale study, but it does offer a clue into how the brain bases of autism in females are possibly different from males.

A more sophisticated approach in the exploration of potential sex differences is to link genetic profiles to brain profiles. It is possible, for example, to look at variations in the genes that determine receptor sites for hormones and compare them with variations in resting-state functional connectivity in the brain. A study in 2020 investigated the relationship between variants of the receptor gene for oxytocin (OXTR), a hormone linked to social behaviour, and resting-state functional connectivity in key hubs of the brain's reward network, in females and males with and without autism.[31] In autistic females, higher prevalence of OXTR anomalies was linked to increased connectivity within social behaviour networks, whereas in males the atypical hormone receptor profile was linked to *decreased* connectivity. Which looks as if an autism-related suspect gene is having different effects in the brains of females and males.

Now that we can get a full profile of an individual's genome, we can pinpoint all the anomalies in genes that have been linked with autism and generate a risk score, and then compare that risk score with other characteristics. One such study, in 2022, showed that the higher the risk score in autistic males, the greater the connectivity between sensory processing and reward processing centres in the brain and the greater their problems with repetitive and restrictive behaviours.[32] Autistic females who had equivalent risk scores did not show this association, which could be interpreted as another teasing clue about some kind of protective effect at work.

The notion of the female protective effect initially arose when the male spotlight was firmly switched on. It had been an accepted fact that more males than females were autistic so it seemed to follow that there must be some kind of protective buffer in place, with the source undetermined. Certainly, the greater genetic hit evident in those girls that did pass the diagnostic threshold, as well as hints of greater numbers of brain anomalies, supported this idea. However, that is not the only possible interpretation. Evidence of a male bias in the diagnostic process might suggest that girls were not 'protected' from being diagnosed by their biology, but by the fact that the construction and delivery of the tests meant that they had to be considerably worse than their male counterparts before it was accepted that they, too, were on the spectrum. As is usually the case, there is probably a grain of truth in both these arguments, with both entangled in the road to an autism diagnosis.

But the fact still remains that, currently, autism is defined by a set of behaviours and not, as yet, by any measurable biological characteristics, genetic or neurological. So it might be more fruitful to make behaviour the starting point, even though we are actually hoping to find the answer to autism in the brain.

There are two ways to study the link between autistic brains and autistic behaviour. There is the inside-out approach we have followed in this chapter, where you find out as much as you can about the brain characteristics of autistic individuals and see if you can spot the difference between their brains and those of neurotypicals. And there is the outside-in approach, where you focus on all those defining behavioural characteristics of autism and see if you can track them back to their 'source' in the brain.

We should turn, then, to our outside-in approach. Let's focus on autism's differences and difficulties and see if we can track them back into the brain. We know that social behaviour is a core problem for autistic individuals, and we now know that this may well be where we find some insights into why autistic females have been overlooked for so long. Their characteristic camouflaging behaviour seems to suggest that they have a different attitude towards social interaction from what we have seen in the traditional, male-based picture of autism. And it actually adds an additional spin on the female protective effect story – it may be their complex masking behaviour that is preventing them from being diagnosed. So, exploring the brain bases of camouflaging as an atypical pattern of autistic behaviour, more common in females, may offer up some useful clues.

In the last fifteen years or so, social cognitive neuroscientists have been mapping the key networks in the brain that underpin perhaps the most complex aspect of human behaviour, being social. As we have seen, clinicians and psychologists have also been working hard at putting together a much more nuanced picture of the social difficulties that are at the core of the autism experience, including explorations of sex and gender differences. Linking these two areas of research together could well offer the best insights yet into the world of autism.

CHAPTER 6

ON BEING SOCIAL

THE BELIEF THAT AUTISM IS A BIOLOGICALLY DETERMINED, brain-based condition was part of its definition from early days. Kanner explicitly stated that the children he was studying were born without the necessary brain and behaviour mechanisms to become social beings: "These children have come into the world without the innate ability to form the usual, biologically provided, affective contact with people."[1]

As we saw in part 1, psychologists studying autism have addressed the need for a more nuanced understanding of what the broad-brush concept of 'social communication difficulties' means in the everyday life of an autistic person. We have a clearer view of how difficulties with social actions such as maintaining eye contact, observing rules of social distance, and turn-taking can negatively impact social interaction. Interpretation of autistic personal testimonies have highlighted issues such as 'belongingness' and the powerful fear of rejection, and the overwhelming anxiety that can accompany social engagement or even its anticipation. Principally due to such personal testimonies, there is greater appreciation of the impact that autism can have on developing the sense of identity that has been put at the heart of being social – if you need to know where you belong, you need to know who 'you' are. Most of all, 'masking' has itself been unmasked: we are aware of the elaborate camouflaging rituals that can be an exhausting and damaging part of social life for many autistic individuals.

We have a better behavioural framework, then, to guide brain-imaging research in its exploration of the autistic brain and its difficulties with 'affective contact with people'. What does it mean to be social and how does the brain do it?

OUR SOCIAL BRAINS

Kanner's reference to an inborn, biologically provided skill of connecting with other people was remarkably prescient. Only in the last twenty years or so has there been a concerted effort in neuroscience to try and understand the neural underpinnings of social cognition, the various mental steps we have to take in order to navigate the complexities of social interactions with other people. Using an ingenious range of tasks and fMRI scanners, an intricate network of old and new brain structures has been revealed.[2]

Once brain imaging became more freely available to research labs as well as hospitals and clinics the earliest focus was on how the human brain produced those skills that were supposedly uniquely human, such as language and imagination, and artistic and scientific creativity. The emphasis was almost wholly on the individual owners of such skills, and what parts of their brains were responsible for, say, their linguistic abilities or memory powers. But, more recently, there has been a shift away from cognitive achievements in single humans to a search for an understanding of what it is that makes humans social, why and how we form networks, gather together in like-minded 'tribes', solve problems collaboratively. Social behaviour involves an awareness of social scripts and social norms – knowing how to follow unspoken social rules and observe invisible social rituals, avoiding social mistakes and the painful social emotions of embarrassment or shame, or the misery of social rejection.[3] It requires that we all become 'mind-readers', that we should not only have a handle on our own portfolio of knowledge or thoughts or beliefs, we should also be able to infer or predict what our fellow human beings know or think or believe, and adjust our behaviour accordingly. This way we can ensure that we fit in, or realize that it might be time to bail out and move on, or to gauge whether, on meeting someone new, this 'other' should be welcomed into our own in-group or whether they are an out-group member and should be ostracized or rejected.

As we saw earlier, developmental psychologists have shown that babies arrive in their world with well-tuned social radar and are able to pick up important social cues right from the beginning. And by three months old they can pick up on highly sophisticated social cues, such as those flagged by eye contact. If someone is looking at you, you have their attention, right? But if they are looking elsewhere, they are ignoring you or (hard to believe) they have found something more interesting to look at. Three-month-old babies can get very agitated if they are confronted with someone who is not looking directly at them (especially if it's their mother or primary carer). So not only are they aware of this 'other' person, they are aware that the other is not interacting with them as they should. There are other stages of picking up on social cues, such as joint attention, where someone's pointing finger can alert you to the fact that they want to share some information with you, to look where they are looking. Or you might realize that if someone is looking fixedly at something, it might be worth your while to have a look too.

Social and clinical psychology research has demonstrated our powerful need to belong to social groups, and has shown how much our self-esteem is entangled with social success, revealing the damaging consequences of negative social experiences such as rejection, ostracism, and loneliness. Neuroscience researchers are starting to map out the brain circuits underpinning social behaviour.

So social cognitive neuroscience is emerging as the ideal forum for our outside-in approach to understanding autism. How do we brain imagers go about spotting the brain's engagement with our social world?

Brain imaging and bony elbows

If you volunteer as a participant in a social brain-imaging study of mine, you could find yourself lying in the brain scanner being asked to pick out those phrases that best describe yourself from a list of options.[4] These might include 'People respect me', 'I can be trusted', or 'People find me difficult to talk to'. The source of the brain activity associated with such musings could then be linked to the processing of your self-identity or self-image (formally referred to as 'self-referential processing').[5] In order to separate this kind of self-identity from your physical characteristics, you might be asked to agree or disagree with statements such as 'I have bony elbows'. (This does, of course, assume that your bony elbows are not a key part of your self-identity!) But what about 'other' processing? Being social invariably involves understanding other people. So you may be asked to agree or disagree with matching statements about your nominated best friend or

Harry Potter or even the queen – 'My best friend is easy to talk to', or 'Harry Potter can be trusted'. And yes, you might need to comment on the statement, 'The queen has bony elbows'. Or you'd have to choose from a list of groups you think you definitely belong to – eco-warrior, tennis player, football supporter, Democrat voter, for example. Or those that you most definitely don't identify with, such as social media influencer, potholer (or spelunker if you hail from the US), or tax evader. Feel free to add to either list.

As well as tracking the people-focussed aspects of social cognition in your brain, I might be interested in your understanding of nonverbal social cues, such as the processing of faces, especially including emotional expressions. For example, I might study how you respond to a direct or averted eye gaze when you watch a video of someone supposedly talking to you (How long does it take you to shout 'over here' at the television when the weather forecaster is looking at the wrong camera?).

These kinds of tasks will activate one of the newest, evolutionarily speaking, parts of your brain – the prefrontal cortex, with tiny differences showing up between the 'self' and 'other', and 'in-group' and 'out-group' responses. It would appear that part of the function of the newly emerging frontal lobes in the human brain is to keep a register of useful social information, acquiring and updating a social knowledge store. It turns out that there is a brain network focussed on monitoring this social store called the default mode network. It becomes active when you are not task-focussed but just mentally idling. When you are sitting idly gazing out of the window, thinking of nothing in particular, or daydreaming, your brain is actually pretty active. (You might like to ponder how much of your daydreaming involves thinking about yourself, or yourself in relation to other people, or in imaginary social scenarios.)

As well as having the cognitive wherewithal to be social, you need motivation to be social. You must *want* to belong to social groups, to engage with others, to actively engage in what is called 'prosocial behaviour'. Back to the scanner, where you find yourself engaged in depressing, self-esteem puncturing tasks devised by yet another social cognitive neuroscientist. This might involve you in scenarios involving social rejection, such as Tinder-type tasks, where you have to respond enthusiastically to pictures of potential partners, only to be shown that each of those potential partners has swiped left when they saw your picture. Or watch your image being awarded a low score on a measure of physical attractiveness.[6] This will (understandably) activate the emotional coding parts of your brain, particularly a part of the brain called the insula, buried deep within the cerebral cortex, which plays a crucial role in understanding and experiencing emotions.

Brain responses to social rejection, and their sources, are very similar to those associated with actual physical pain.[7] This provides important clues that negative social experiences may be powerful driving forces in shaping human behaviour. Being social, satisfying the need to belong, can be as fundamentally motivating as the need to survive, the need to find food and water, and the need to mate. The brain mechanisms activated by social rejection, as well as being linked to real pain, have also been shown to be associated with severe cases of depression, as well as chronic eating disorders. The need to belong, and the consequences of being rejected, is clearly an important force in human behaviour.

More cheeringly, you might take part in a task where you have a high success rate, each triumph eliciting a bright smiley emoji.[8] This will activate your striatum, a part of the limbic system, the brain's reward centre. The striatum is evolutionarily primitive but highly active even in today's more complex social world – especially when confronted with rewarding or pleasurable experiences, such as social approval or acceptance. Together with the insula, mentioned previously, the striatum is a key part of the brain's salience network, which makes sure we are paying attention to the right information at the right time.

So we have a sophisticated storage system for high-level social information, such as a sense of self or the difference between in-groups and out-groups, and a primitive but powerful coding system, which will tag social information, or the outcomes of social events, as positive or negative. We also need a social regulation system that can use this information to steer us through the complicated rules of social interaction, away from social faux pas, and towards social acceptance and a sense of belonging.

To help us brain imagers find this social regulation system, you might find yourself staring at series of brightly coloured shapes on a screen and, every now and then, a face.[9] You have to press a button as fast as possible if you see a face (which counts as a social target). Or you gaze at a series of faces and every now and then a coloured shape appears, requiring a button press. These kinds of studies, sometimes called 'go/no-go' tasks, have shown that we normally respond faster to social stimuli, such as faces, than to neutral stimuli, such as abstract shapes, and that a part of the brain called the anterior cingulate cortex (ACC) appears to be in charge of activating this speedy response.

The ACC is neatly situated between the newer information processing centres found in the prefrontal areas and the older emotional processing centres deep in the brain. As a result, it is well-placed to match social information with any 'go' or 'no-go' tags, and to initiate the best sort of response. In another, more sophisticated, go/no-go test involving the ACC, you might be shown a series of faces, almost all expressionless, and told NOT to respond to any that were happy or sad.[10] This is actually quite hard, as you will have to override what seems to be an automatic response to anything that carries social information. The ACC again appears to be in charge of this kind of social conflict monitoring. It has been described as a kind of inner critic, or inner limiter, making sure we focus on the things that matter (and act accordingly) and ignore those that don't.

These contemporary studies have identified those brain networks that underpin some of the rules that individuals need to follow in order to be successfully social, the types of social 'etiquette' with which autistic individuals struggle. But there is another aspect of being social that takes us back to the early days of psychological theories of autism – the skills of understanding other people, or 'mind-reading' (or the lack of such skills, known as 'mindblindness', which we encountered in chapter 3). Social judgements about how we view ourselves and how we view others – and, of course, how they view us – are sufficiently important that we have dedicated brain areas that allow us to make judgements and evaluations about others in social contexts. But it turns out that we need more than just a mental catalogue of social information in order to mix with other people. We need to get inside their minds.

HUMAN BEINGS AS MIND-READERS

To behave as social beings, we must tackle the complexities of not only knowing ourselves, but getting to know other people and understand how they behave. As well as picking up on basic social information flagged by others – do they look like us and so are more likely to behave like us, for example – we need to know much, much more about them. It is not exaggeration to say that we need to be able to get inside the mind of anyone we might want, or need, or even be forced, to interact with. We have to acquire some kind of insight into how they might interact with us or other people, what their – obviously invisible – inner thoughts or intentions or wishes might be. This is known as having a 'theory of mind'.[11]

To be successful mind-readers we need to be able to interpret a whole range of social cues – facial expressions, tone of voice, perhaps gestures and other types of body language. You might add some previous knowledge of the kind of person you are dealing with – are they a peaceable type who will be happy to go with the flow, or a firebrand who will argue with you just for the sake of it? You might even add some stereotypes into your social sleuthing kit – this person is female so is more likely to be empathic and collegial; this person is male, so may be assertive and independent.

It turns out that this sophisticated, socially important ability to work out what is in someone else's mind, and how that will affect their behaviour, emerges at a surprisingly young age. We know this thanks to a task developed by psychologists Heinz Wimmer and Josef Perner in 1983, the so-called Sally-Anne task.[12]

Children are shown two puppet dolls, Sally and Anne, with two containers – a box and a basket. Sally puts a ball in the basket and goes away, out of sight. Anne then moves Sally's ball into the box. Sally comes back. The children are asked where Sally will look for her ball.

Children who have developed a theory of mind (usually between three and four years old) will say that Sally will look for her ball in the basket because they have 'read' Sally's mind and realized that Sally won't know Anne moved the ball, so will look for the ball where she, Sally, left it. Children whose theory of mind hasn't developed yet (usually under three years old) will tell you that Sally will look for the ball in the box because that is where they, the observers, last saw it. Egocentrically, they don't take account of the fact that Sally won't know her ball has been moved.

Innovative research initiated by Simon Baron-Cohen and Uta and Chris Frith suggested that difficulties with mind-reading could be at the heart of the social difficulties characteristic of autism.[13] Up to 80 per cent of autistic children struggle with theory of mind tests. And these struggles continue into adulthood – the phrase 'just put yourself in their shoes' remains puzzling to many autistic adults (aside from the difficulties caused by a tendency for over-literal interpretation of such instructions). I once got embroiled in a lengthy debate with two autistic males who were scornfully dismissing the notion of empathy – 'How on earth could you get inside someone else's head to know how they were feeling?'

Here, then, is another template of human social behaviour that brain imagers could use to investigate both typical and atypical social skills. Having developed theory-of-mind tasks for the scanner, it became evident that there is another specialized network that is activated by all forms of mind-reading.[14]

Given the role of understanding other people in being social, the network involved in the theory of mind is, understandably, closely entangled with the social brain network and the social reward system. The ventromedial prefrontal cortex is part of the brain network involved in our sense of self, knowing our own mind. When reading other minds, it is commonly the adjacent dorsomedial prefrontal cortex that is primarily involved. So a 'they-don't-know-that-I-know-what-they-don't-know' theory-of-mind–type dialogue is supported by minutely distinct, but efficiently close, parts of the brain. The dorsomedial prefrontal cortex is widely involved in a range of social processing skills, such as monitoring the outcomes of social exchanges, coding the characteristics of those involved, and registering any action patterns associated with the exchange. So this part of the brain would be involved in tracking the high-level, more abstract aspects of the social world. Here you will see the effects of irony and sarcasm, where what is said is not necessarily what is meant; of insights into people's emotions by looking at their eyes; of reading personality traits; of guessing at intentions.

Then there are the two-way exchanges between the temporal lobes, centrally involved in many aspects of memory (such as the 'what happened before?' type of information, or 'what did that particular type of emotional expression mean?', or 'what was meant by that particular tone of voice?'), and the junction between the temporal lobes and the parietal lobes (helpfully called the temporo-parietal junction), which co-ordinates many of the brain's sensory and perceptual processing systems. This is where useful social cues or clues will be processed, such as working out other people's mental states, or processing different intonations of speech.

As noted earlier, the theory-of-mind brain, or mentalizing, network is closely entangled with the social brain and the salience networks, with the hard-working ACC at their heart. Together they work to ensure the success of social exchanges, updating your sense of self. You might think, 'That was great – I seem to get on well with people like that', reflecting on the success of your mind-reading. And, 'I could see they were interested in what I was saying', coding the characteristics of those involved. And 'It helped that we supported the same football team', and registering any action patterns associated with the exchange – 'I'm glad I shook hands with them all'.

Interactions within and between these networks underpin all aspects of social behaviour, from the simple recognition of a friend's face (with the appropriate 'pleased to see you' expression generated on your own face) to the different phases of affective and cognitive empathy, to feeling someone else's distress, perhaps, and understanding what to do about it.

Neuroscientists have provided a robust framework with which to explore the brain bases of social behaviour.[15] They have found ways of tracking the interplay between the social knowledge stores in the prefrontal cortex and the social-motivational centres, involving emotional coding structures such as the amygdala, the insula, and the striatum.[16] They have shown how these link up to our mind-reading centres, helping us predict how those around us will interact with us. They have also characterized our social regulation system, based on the ACC, helping us successfully navigate the nuances of social scripts, enabling us to produce the socially appropriate patterns of behaviour.[17] When we get it right, there's a thumbs up from our salience/reward system; when we get it wrong, that's stored away for future reference.

All these networks and systems maximize our chances of finding our tribe and fitting in. Using this framework, we should be able to investigate what it is about social interaction and social communication that autistic individuals find so challenging.

In the last chapter, we looked at what geneticists and developmental neuroscientists could tell us about why, when, and how the autistic brain is different from the typical brain. The bigger picture showed that we are looking at a fundamental alteration in the brain's wiring blueprint that could initially disrupt basic, localized sensory processes but, crucially, have downstream consequences for the formation of the higher-level networks spread throughout the brain. Is there any evidence of this kind of disruption in social networks in the autistic brain?

Once the autism neuroscience research community began focussing on the connectivity between social brain networks, rather than looking at individual components, substantial progress began to be made, albeit with one sadly predictable failing. One study of twenty-nine participants showed lower levels of connectivity, particularly involving connections to the prefrontal areas, and to the emotion control centres such as the amygdala. The weaker the connections, the higher the levels of social impairment shown by the autistic group.[18] Of the twenty-nine participants, only one was female.

It was a small-scale study but was backed up by later findings. In 2013, Simon Baron-Cohen's Cambridge group looked at specific social brain networks, such as the default mode network (the self-reference, daydreaming network or DMN), and the salience network.[19] These showed reduced connectivity in autistic brains, not only within each network hub, but also between them. Again, this was a small-scale study with fifteen ASD participants – in this case, *all* of them were male.

A more sophisticated study in 2020 looked at dynamic connectivity, the extent to which different parts of key networks become activated at the same time, a measure of their efficiency.[20] Here the focus was on the salience network, which includes both the insula and the ACC. This time there were slightly more autistic participants, but the cohort was still rather biased, with sixty-four boys and eleven girls, aged between six and thirteen years. Patterns of co-activation were significantly weaker in the ASD group. There was an apologetic mention of the male-female imbalance.

A picture of how the miswiring of the autistic brain impacts social brain function was emerging. But it was almost entirely limited to the male autistic brain. It could be that this miswiring problem was indeed sex-independent, caused by misinformation in the autism genome, exerting its effect on the brain irrespective of the sex of its owner. This conclusion would have been acceptable if there was strong evidence that social-behavioural problems in autistic males and autistic females were pretty much the same. However, the first half of this book should have convinced you otherwise! Increasing evidence about a distinctive difference in social motivation, possibly illustrated by a tendency to mask or camouflage autistic behaviours, indicates that investigations into the brain bases of autistic behaviours *should* include exploration of sex/gender differences as well. We shall turn to this in the next chapter, but first, we need to delve into a revolutionary advance in our understanding of the brain – and how it impacts our search for autism's neurological origins.

YOUR BRAIN AS A PREDICTION MACHINE

Much early brain research viewed the brain as a relatively passive recipient of information to be processed, coding those things that demanded attention as they arrived, and relatively rapidly switching off responses to those that didn't. A newer model of how our brains work and what they are for is based on the idea that the brain is like a guessing machine.[21] Effectively, it makes predictions about future outcomes of incoming data (rather like a weather-forecasting system), producing generic 'short cuts' to save the time and effort involved in analyzing every new event from scratch. These predictions are called 'establishing a prior' (making a bet) about incoming information. If the 'guess' turns out to be wrong, the brain will then signal an error and reconfigure its instructions to make sure the mistake is not repeated in the future.

The aim of predictive coding is to economize on brain activity. If the prior is successful – say a sound signals the beginning of a familiar melody, or your cheerful response to a smiling face is well received – then minimal further processing will be required. If, however, a discordant note follows, or your cheerful response is met with a punch in the face, then the signalling of the 'prediction error' will flag up the need to search for the next best guess. On average, priors will be fairly general or 'good enough', so an approximate match will do and your brain will signal that what you did worked out fine. If this is the case, next time you should be able to get away with paying little or no attention. But if your brain creates predictions that overspecify what should come next, then even the minutest deviation could be registered as an error and you'll constantly be returning to the drawing board to switch off the error-generating system.

The updating and resetting is effortlessly seamless. Information from a multitude of different sources is efficiently analyzed and combined, or discarded as necessary. The process is continuous and dynamic, with networks of different brain areas being coupled and uncoupled over millisecond timescales.

In 2012, psychologists Elizabeth Pellicano and David Burr suggested that this kind of model of brain function could be useful in understanding some of the sensory and perceptual anomalies associated with autism.[22] For example, some autistic people show less susceptibility to visual illusions, high levels of performance on visual search tasks, and a stunning memory for visual detail. In predictive coding terms, autistic brains could be establishing minutely detailed 'priors', great for hugely accurate assessments of the immediate event but then constantly at the mercy of the siren sounds of prediction errors.

How to measure this predictive coding system at work, or track a faulty one? Early brain-imaging techniques were not capable of tracking the where and when, or the to and fro, of this exquisitely detailed guessing game, but newer approaches are beginning to capture what is going on.

Much of such newer approaches revolve around the reading of different 'frequencies' of brain signals. Communication in the brain involves continuous electrochemical exchanges between eighty-six billion or so nerve cells, within and between brain structures. The resulting electrical signals from the synchronized activity of large groups of neurons can be picked up by various brain-imaging techniques and then matched to different physical or mental states (such as sleep or daydreaming) or particular types of behaviour. These signals have different frequencies, like radio signals, determined by the rate at which nerve cells are firing. Neuroscientists have discovered that different brain structures and networks may be associated with particular frequencies, such as the very slow waves coming from deep within the brain that accompany sleep.

Many people are familiar with the term 'alpha rhythm', a particular brain wave frequency that appears and disappears with variations in attention and became popular in the 1980s heyday of biofeedback, with promises of 'effortless creativity' and 'comfort, peace, happiness, and harmony' once you learned to enhance your brain's alpha activity. But there are many different frequencies, from the very slow delta waves that accompany sleep to the much faster gamma waves associated with high-level brain function, such as perception, memory, and attention.

The research group I was working with aimed to use brain-imaging techniques to track the appearance and disappearance of these frequencies across the whole brain, not just from one fixed location.[23] This would give us real-time insights into how the brain creates predictions and tweaks them. We saw how one area of the brain resonates at a particular frequency when some information arrives, like a tuning-fork, and then feeds this forward to other areas that also resonate at this frequency – rather like different parts of an orchestra playing the same part of a tune. With input from other parts of the brain coming in – perhaps as the result of an error being signalled – we might be able to watch a different frequency feeding back to the original area, signalling a successful harmony or, alternatively, an unsuccessful discord. We hoped this investigation would give us a much better handle on the efficiency or otherwise of our brains and how they handle the experiences our worlds are throwing at us.

To show you how we tested this, I need to introduce you to another scanning task.

ZAP THE ALIENS

Our young participants, autistic or neurotypical, would sit quietly in a scanner, cheerily playing our Zap the Aliens game. For each trial, as soon as a virtual spaceship porthole opened on their screen, they would ready themselves for the appearance of their next target. If it was an alien, then they were instructed to press the trigger to blast the alien. If it was an astronaut, they would have to hold fire. (We did try to develop a less gung ho version, where you could feed the astronaut a cookie or withhold it from the alien, but that failed to hold the children's interest for long enough. 'Arming' them resulted in rapt attention and enthusiastic engagement.) In some respects, the game was an irrelevance. What we were actually interested in was their brain's response to the clicking sound that accompanied the appearance of the porthole and the stark checkerboard pattern that surrounded it. We knew that, at the beginning, there would be a 'what's that?' response when the porthole first appeared on the screen or the clicks played out through the headphones. As the game progressed, we predicted that this response would rapidly diminish with a 'nothing to see here . . . no need to log this . . . carry on as you are' response. Their brain had 'established a prior', or made a successful guess about what was likely to come next.

We could just have sat our participants in the scanner and flashed checkerboard patterns at them or bombarded them with clicking sounds over and over (and over) again to collect enough data to see what was happening in the brain. Indeed, we did this with our heroic colleagues who helped us develop this test of brain reactivity. But it was found to be really, really boring and people quickly became fidgety, fell asleep, or just kept missing their cues (or all of the above). We were hoping to try out this task on younger participants, both neurotypical and autistic, and guessed there would be no chance of persuading them to spend any length of time 'mindlessly' staring at patterns or listening to clicks. So we came up with the idea of embedding this meaningless train of information in our Zap the Aliens game.

Did the task give us a useful measure of predictive coding at work? Fortunately, yes.[24] We showed that, in the typically developing brain, there was a pattern of gamma waves flowing forward from the sensory areas to the frontal lobes, gradually ebbing as the game went on. This was followed by backward-washing alpha waves, from frontal lobes back to the sensory areas, which we characterized as a 'pay attention, check this out' message, morphing to a calming 'nothing new to see here, no mistakes made, carry on as you are'.

But the brain activity was not the same in our autistic participants. The 'pay attention' message carried by the feedforward gamma wave carried on at the same level of intensity, but was not followed by the calming, no-error message carried by the feedback alpha waves.[25] The arrival of each stimulus activated a rather exaggerated 'what's that?' response that in turn continuously activated the brain's error logging systems. A highly efficient switch-on response unfortunately matched with an inefficient switch-off one. The study showed that the brain of an autistic individual could pay highly focussed attention to just about everything in its environment, but was less able to register what didn't matter, what could be ignored. Effectively, it was less capable at discerning spam from message, at learning what was salient and what wasn't, and how to behave accordingly. And each of these problems could be linked to the atypical pathways in the social brain that neuroscience is starting to track.

One of the consequences of a 'prediction error' being flagged is that the brain has to activate a warning system – a reboot or a rethink. Most of the time this is an automatic, unconscious process, a smooth adjustment to ongoing activity, a quick rerouting to a safer outcome. However, an alarm will have been triggered – maybe a quiet nudge that a bit more attention is required – a bit like a suggestion to the driver of an autonomous car that perhaps they should take the wheel for a bit. But suppose your alarm system was permanently set to a maximum 'code red' setting: any variation in the expectation established by your prior – whether it was what your breakfast should smell like, or the route you take to school, or a flickering fluorescent light in your office – anything would set your heart racing, your palms sweating, your stomach churning. And it might even get to the point that these things didn't even have to actually happen. Just the anticipation of what *might* happen, what sounds you *might* encounter, what social rules you *might* break would be enough to trigger your alarm.

Paradoxically, this is, of course, what predictive coding is all about – establishing a prior to allow you to anticipate the future. But, in order to be effective, it has to be flexible, and an acceptable margin of error should take into account the fact that it is operating in a relatively uncertain world. 'Good enough' will do. But a badly programmed coding system – as in autism – can set you up with a problematic prior. If it overspecifies what should come next, demanding an exact match, then any tiny deviation will set off your alarm. If on the other hand, the to-and-fro messages are distorted by a noisy system, and you've got no clear prediction of what comes next, then you may well be stuck in high-alert mode.[26]

How might this play out in the social world? As opposed to a swift check of ongoing world events, effortlessly decoded and recoded for predicted outcomes, with the appropriate action programme immediately activated, the autistic brain seems to go back to basics, exhaustively (and exhaustingly) logging every tiny incoming detail, constantly flagging up panic-inducing mismatch warnings, never allowing the formation of useful cognitive short cuts. Every sight or sound is flagged as 'new, possibly dangerous' and magnified as a consequence (think of constantly crashing percussion instruments).

If you think about it, much of social behaviour has to do with anticipation.[27] We've already talked about mind-reading, almost all of which is anticipating or making predictions about how other people will react to you, or matching past experiences with the social situation you are currently confronting. In order words, it involves establishing a prior and flagging up prediction errors.

We have seen how the activities of the social brain act a bit like a social GPS system, tracking social data and directing our social behaviour accordingly. Working in conjunction with some kind of predictive system based on previous interactions, we are normally safely guided through the intricacies of the social world. But any glitch in this system and its workings could make it a puzzlingly unpredictable place. It would make other people an insoluble mystery and any form of social contact a source of anxiety and stress.

The neuroscience community has started to pinpoint how the social brain struggles in autistic individuals. But up to now, the picture has been incomplete. The clinicians and psychologists have opened our eyes with respect to just how different the traditional, Kanner-type autism phenotype, mainly true of males, is from the chameleon-type autism phenotype, mainly true of females. The neuroscience community needs to start exploring where these differences might come from, and whether the distinctiveness of what is going on at the behavioural level is matched by the distinctiveness of what is happening in the brain.

CHAPTER 7

KANNER BRAINS AND CHAMELEON BRAINS

A FEMALE SPOTLIGHT?

MY QUESTIONS TO AUTISTIC FEMALES ABOUT WHAT THEY might like to know from a brain scientist led to lots of requests for brain explanations of the everyday difficulties of being autistic. There was near universal agreement that their brains worked differently, and a flattering fascination when I held forth about predictive coding and salience networks (no, really). I explained that it was unlikely that brain researchers would ever find a handy autism-specific marker in the brain, but that we might find out the basis of the various difficulties they experienced. The overwhelming issue for most of the females I spoke to was of their wish to fit in with other people, to be able to 'effortlessly socialize' and not be held hostage by the overwhelming anxiety caused by difficulties in the outside world. When I asked what worried them most, 'people changing plans' easily came top, with various versions of 'not having any friends' frequently mentioned.

This chapter explores what research has been done to date to address these issues. And, more to the point, what remains to be done.

DSM-5 tells us that a key defining feature of autism is 'persistent deficits in social communications and interactions'.[1] Traditionally that has mapped onto the stereotypical idea of isolated, socially awkward males, who seem somehow set apart from day-to-day social life. As Kanner noted, they seem to lack the fundamental human motivation to make contact with other people, to belong to a social world.

However, we have seen that a significant proportion of the autism community, most of whom are female, do not fit into this picture of autism. They certainly seem to have difficulties with social interactions, but these appear to arise for different reasons. They do not seem to lack the motivation to belong – indeed their personal accounts suggest that they experience belonging as a hugely powerful need, so strong that they desperately try to hide their autistic traits. Nevertheless, they seem to lack the necessary skill set to make it happen.

In the first half of the book, we saw how this newer conception of autism is finally being unpacked by behavioural scientists. But are neuroscientists following suit? If they are looking for problems in the social brain, are they looking in the right place?

One question to ask is whether any differences in the brains of autistic females might be an extension of differences in the brains of all females. We already know that there is very little evidence of differences in brain structures between males and females.

However, we need to avoid the traditional tendency to think of sex-related differences in the brain just in terms of structures or the brain's hardware. If we really want to understand the relationship between our brains and a particular aspect of our behaviour, such as being social, then we need to map the brain activation patterns associated with whatever skill we are interested in.

You may recall, way back in chapter 2, there was an update on the centuries-old female/male brain debate, where a team from Chicago, led by Lise Eliot, had painstakingly picked through thirty years' worth of brain-imaging research to see how well it supported the notion that there were two (and only two) different kinds of brains that were measurably distinct.[2] It didn't, as flagged by the pithy title 'Dump the "Dimorphism"'. This survey did not relate only to structures in the brain; it also looked at patterns of brain activation associated with different types of cognitive or emotional skills that were stereotypically either female or male. One set of skills included various types of emotional processing, firmly embedded in theories of autistic behaviour. Eliot's team collated all the studies looking at sex differences in brain activation during tasks involving emotional processing – seven meta-analyses comprising 410 studies in all. The conclusion was that, overall, men and women activate the same neural structures when processing emotions. We should also recall the gigantic, worldwide survey of sex differences in empathy, using self-report measures and the RMET, which we talked about in chapter 3. Statistical comparisons were interpreted as evidence of what looked like a universal female advantage in empathy. But there was a huge amount of variability and the differences were 'vanishingly' small.[3]

In typical populations, then, there is little or no evidence of sex differences in the brain bases of the types of behaviour that seem particularly problematic for at least part of the autism community.

This would indicate that, if such differences are found in the autistic population (assuming anyone is looking), it demonstrates an autism-specific influence at work, and is not just an extension of something we might expect to see in typical brains.

WHERE HAVE ALL THE GIRLS GONE?

We know that females who should be eligible for inclusion in autism research are being vigorously rejected by the so-called gold standard tests for autism. This clearly seems to have had an impact on neuroscience research too. If you recall, a survey in 2021 of over 1,400 brain-imaging studies of autism showed that over 30 per cent of such studies used only male participants.[4] The ratios varied depending on what was being measured – the ratio of males:females in the structural studies was about 6:1; in task-related fMRI studies it was about 15:1; and resting state studies came in at 9:1. So very few of these studies even matched the traditional 4:1 ratio, which we now know probably does not reflect the true proportion of males and females in the autism community.

But the problem doesn't stop there. As autism is such a varied condition, you really need to run studies with hundreds, if not thousands, of participants in order to detect any meaningful differences in the noise that is invariably autism data. This is more than any single lab or research group could ever hope to recruit. So autism researchers have pooled their resources and shared all their information, including genetic, biochemical, medical, and behavioural profiles, as well as data from as many different brain-imaging studies as were available. These so-called big datasets can then be used by any autism researcher to test out hypotheses, make comparisons, and explore relationships between dozens of different variables.[5] The participants who were recruited into these collectives could also be available for additional research studies, greatly cutting down the labour-intensive aspect of each research group finding and assessing autistic participants for testing.

You will recall that, in chapter 2, I mentioned that in my area, neuroimaging, the ABIDE was launched in 2012, aiming to facilitate the sharing of resting-state fMRI data from individuals with autism. And that I grumpily noted that, in the first version of this initiative, ABIDE I, only 12 per cent of the more than one thousand fMRI resting-state datasets and phenotypic datasets from over 539 diagnosed autistic individuals were female.

A paper published in *Molecular Psychiatry* proudly announced a demonstration of how these data could be used to investigate brain architecture in minute detail.[6] Their enthusiasm was evident: 'ABIDE is expected to accelerate the pace of discovery setting the stage for the next generation of ASD studies. . . . [T]he construction and open release of the ABIDE sample represents a landmark milestone in autism imaging'.

So the showcase demonstration – a hugely useful insight into atypical brain connectivity in autism – analyzed only the data from males. In the paper's closing paragraphs, where the researchers highlighted 'emerging significant themes that merit further study', they discussed controls for IQ differences, and the need to image toddlers and pre-schoolers. Females didn't get a mention.

To be fair, there is an ABIDE II that has collected over one thousand additional datasets and the number of ASD females has risen to 15 per cent.[7] The coverage of this newer dataset does elaborate on the problem of heterogeneity in its samples and acknowledges the problem of 'sex-related differences . . . [that] have been generally ignored in the ASD imaging literature due to the markedly higher prevalence of males with ASD and the tendency of single sites to exclude or minimally represent females'.

Several more big datasets have been created. The Simons Foundation Autism Research Initiative (SFARI) launched SPARK (Simons Foundation Powering Autism Research for Knowledge) in April 2016.[8] Aiming for fifty thousand individuals, calculated to be the number needed to carry out meaningful genetic investigations, by 2022 they had data from over 130,000 autistic individuals, together with parents and unaffected siblings. There were over 97,000 autistic males and nearly 35,000 autistic females, reflecting a male:female ratio of 2.79:1, so definitely an improvement on early ABIDE days! In Europe there was the EU-AIMS (European Union–Autism Interventions–a Multi-centre Study) project, part of which comprised a longitudinal project (Longitudinal European Autism Project, or LEAP).[9] A total of 437 autistic individuals were signed up for the study. They were specifically recruited with a male:female ratio of 3:1, so the male spotlight is still at work, but again with better representation than ABIDE I.

One significant aspect of these autism datasets was that eligibility for inclusion almost invariably involved confirmation via the use of the gold standard ADOS and/or ADI tests. You may recall the MIT group that we met in chapter 2 who identified what they called the leaky pipeline problem with respect to recruiting (and then losing) autistic females from their own recruitment programme.[10] They also surveyed several large, publicly available autism datasets. They found that where ADOS had been used to determine inclusion, the male:female ratio was of the order of 7:1. Where the datasets had relied on community diagnoses or screening from whole populations, the ratios varied from 0.68 to 1.8 to 1. Therefore, any research using such datasets is likely to be deeply flawed. And indeed it is.

THE SOCIAL BRAIN IN AUTISM: KANNER OR CHAMELEON?

Neuroimaging studies undertaken before the establishment of big datasets (however skewed) were generally carried out on small numbers of participants, sometimes a few dozen, or maybe just into three figures. Even if a statistically significant finding was discovered, in populations as widely varying as autistic groups, it was likely to be quite small and quite possibly wasn't replicated in other, similar studies. But once a substantial number of studies had been carried out, it was possible to perform what is called a meta-analysis, which is a survey of all such studies where the results could be combined to see what consistent patterns might emerge. In other words, through using meta-analyses, we can more reliably pinpoint where the differences between autistic brains and neurotypical brains might lie. Sometimes, a helpful technique called activation likelihood estimation (ALE) can also be applied. ALE looks at the co-ordinates in the brain where the significant differences were encountered in each of the studies and pinpoints the overlap. This can give an exact location of those brain areas that are most consistently involved, and acts as strong evidence in support of any model linking brain structures or functions to a particular type of behaviour.

With respect to studies of the social brain, imagers would want to target any parts of the prefrontal cortex that had been linked to social knowledge processing, including the DMN, our self-referencing, daydreaming centre. We would also definitely need to consider the social regulation system – the social GPS tracker – which, if you recall, involves the ACC acting rather like a behavioural go/no-go traffic light system, encouraging social behaviour that has previously resulted in a good outcome, or inhibiting anything that didn't turn out so well.

Another key focus should be on the social reward system, the system that codes social situations as something to be avoided or as something to be sought. Mapping the interplay between the ACC and structures such as the insula and the striatum, as well as the salience network, could not only reveal the brain bases of autism's atypical social behaviour, but provide some clues about the differences between the predominantly male, Kanner-like individuals who are indifferent about social contact and the predominantly female, chameleon-like maskers.

One meta-analysis plus ALE report, published in 2021, collated studies that focussed on the social reward system.[11] This included fMRI-based tasks measuring how quickly a happy face was distinguished from a sad one (sometimes with the faces only partly shown or blurred), or some kind of reward feedback task, where a correct answer could earn a smiley face or an incorrect one a grumpy one.

The conclusions of the survey were clear: autistic participants consistently showed under-activation in the striatum (a key part of the social reward system in the brain). I was intrigued to see if this finding was true of females as well as males. After all, the camouflaging literature had raised the question of why females were putting themselves through such an exhausting exercise in order to fit in or belong. But frustratingly, the summary table of the papers surveyed reported only the total numbers of autistic participants in each of the studies, and didn't give a female/male breakdown. So I had go to each of the twenty-three studies to get my question answered. You can probably now guess what I found.

The papers were published between 2008 and 2020, and the numbers scanned in each study were relatively modest, between eight and thirty-eight. Over 40 per cent of the studies scanned only males. Out of a total across all studies of 434 autistic participants, only fifty-one (11 per cent) were female. This figure was not even representative of the traditional male:female 4:1 claim.

Neither the authors of the survey nor those of any of the papers reviewed felt it necessary to even comment on the fact that they were only (or mainly) looking at males. On the contrary, the authors firmly concluded that the research they had reviewed provided 'robust' evidence for an underactive striatum in reward processing, and highlighted the importance of this evidence in understanding autism. Overall, they suggest that these research findings add up to support a (rather grim) image of autism as a condition of 'diminished pleasure, reduced motivation to acquire rewarding stimuli and less avoidance of punishment'. Somewhat alarmingly, they suggest that, in the future, neurostimulation techniques could be brought into play, to turbocharge the somnolent striatum.

I widened my search to check on other studies looking at the social reward system in autism. They were mainly grouped into six more surveys.[12] In addition to the original one I had looked at, these covered over 120 additional studies, carried out over a thirty-year period between 1990 and 2020. The overall picture from every single one of these surveys was of patterns of underactivity in all or many parts of the social brain or, in one survey, evidence of structural underconnectivity within the social brain network. The narrative around these findings was firmly linked to the Kanner-type autism phenotype, of minimal social interaction, linked to reduced social motivation, arising from a dysfunctional social reward system. These studies looked like a powerful evidence base from which to construct a model of autism in the brain.

Again, I had to go back to each of the original papers to get detailed information about how many males and how many females were involved.[13] Of the more than four thousand participants tested, fewer than 10 per cent were female. Looking at each survey, and averaging across the cohorts from each of the studies reported, the male:female ratios of autistic participants ranged from 27:1 to 6.29:1. Put another way, the percentage of females tested ranged from 13.7 to 3.5 per cent.

Obviously, none of the studies had carried out any sex difference analyses – tricky if only one of your participants is female! The authors of three of the surveys did make passing reference to this in their discussions of the limitations of their review. Rather more concerningly, the studies themselves invariably reported their findings in terms of only 'autism' or 'ASD participants' or 'ASD' youth. Only a small number drew attention to the fact that they didn't look at females at all, again in something of a passing reference at the end of their reports.

It is not hard to see how we arrived at this state of affairs and how, as a researcher, you might rationalize your very skewed group of participants. It was really, really hard to recruit female autistic participants, so you took who you could get. It didn't matter too much if they were all males, because autism is characteristically a male problem so, in fact, testing only males was more likely to yield the answers you were looking for. And if you did include females, there wasn't much evidence that they were different from males, so you could assert that their autism diagnosis was the key measure and their sex did not need to be considered. But, whatever the rationale, for thirty years or more, autism researchers were carefully building a model of autism that was based on only part of the autism community. Clearly, the sex/gender irrelevance model had to be tested.

HERE COME THE GIRLS

In 2017, as part of the US Autism Centers of Excellence network, a multidisciplinary research consortium specifically designed to address issues of sex and gender in autism research was launched.[14] Gender Exploration of Neurogenetics and Development to Advance Autism Research (GENDAAR) combined genetic, neuroimaging, and phenotypical data from well-matched samples of girls and boys with and without ASD. As well as the standard ADOS and ADI assessments, potential participants were also assessed using more focussed tests such as the Social Responsiveness Scale or brief screening tests such as the Childhood Autism Rating Scale. Findings from this programme have added to the emerging body of evidence that 'robust' findings in male autistic participants do not always generalize to females.

An effective avenue of research by the GENDAAR consortium has been the repetition of research previously undertaken on mostly male participants, using new groups of participants that were more balanced in gender. For example, one skewed study from 2010 (on sixteen males) reported diminished neural responses to social rewards, especially in the striatum, consistent with the classic autism phenotype of reduced social motivation.[15] A GENDAAR version of this study recruited thirty-nine girls and forty-three boys.[16] The researchers found that autistic girls displayed *increased* activity in the networks associated with social rewards, compared to autistic boys. These patterns of neural activity would be consistent with a more active social reward system and *higher* levels of social motivation, so certainly inconsistent with the accepted autism phenotype (and with previous neuroimaging findings based only on males). One for the Chameleons?

Other parts of the traditional autism picture have also been challenged. If you recall, atypical sensory responsivity

– hyperreactivity to sights or sounds or smells – was added as a core characteristic of autism in the latest DSM iteration. There are consistent reports that it is more common in autistic females than males. One early study reported increased functional connectivity between the salience network (which helps us identify what is important) and primary sensory processing areas in the brain, and a decrease of connectivity with the prefrontal, social knowledge areas.[17] The explanation was that autistic individuals found sensory data more rewarding than social information, so lacked interest in social cues, allegedly typical autistic behaviour. The autistic cohort in this study comprised twenty-seven males and one female. So not that typical then?

In 2020, members of the GENDAAR consortium looked at this relationship again, this time with sixteen females and thirty-seven males in the autistic cohort.[18] Once again, males showed strong functional connectivity between the salience and the primary sensory networks. The higher their levels of sensory over-responsivity, the stronger this connection. For females, however, sensory over-responsivity was more strongly associated with increased functional connectivity between the salience network and the social regulatory areas, including the prefrontal regions and the ACC.

What behavioural differences might we be looking at here? If sounds and smells and lights are more attention-grabbing, it is difficult to focus on the more subtle social niceties. This would fit in with the traditional picture of autism, where sensory information is much more likely to grab the autistic person's attention (or sensory overload much more likely to elicit social avoidance behaviour). Many a time I have had to wait while autistic participants introduced themselves to my laboratory by sniffing every surface or stroking the chair covers before they said hello to me. However, findings from female autistic participants, whom we know tend to have higher levels of sensory difficulties than males, indicate that their salience system seems to be tied more tightly to social behaviour circuits. How might we reconcile these findings? The authors of the paper suggested that there might be a link to a female autistic tendency to monitor and regulate the behavioural consequences of sensory over-responsivity and avoid social embarrassment. Nearly overwhelmed by sensory input, they nevertheless prioritize suppressing any reaction that might draw attention to themselves or be out of keeping with the social niceties of the situation. So it might be that they focus more on social impression management than do their Kanner counterparts. This notion fits in nicely with our picture of chameleon-like behaviour.

One of the autistic teenagers I talked to describes exactly this sort of experience:

> I hated going to church because the smell of the incense and the sound of the bells filled up my head and made me want to put my hands over my ears and scream and run out of the church. But I knew my Mum and Dad would be angry and embarrassed so I found a way of clenching and unclenching my hands inside my coat sleeves until the noise and the smells stopped. I would have rocked but I knew that would get me into trouble too.

Other sex differences came to light when the GENDAAR consortium examined overall connectivity in the autistic social brain. A 2017 paper summarized sixty-seven different studies of resting state measures of autistic brains.[19] The participants were, again, overwhelmingly male. A key finding was underconnectivity in the DMN, our 'daydreaming' self-referencing control centre. The take-home message from these studies was that this underconnectivity was the brain basis of the 'characteristically' impaired processing of social signals in autism. Six of these studies had no female ASD participants, and females represented only 9.3 per cent of the overall total of these connectivity studies.

The GENDAAR team investigated the same relationship, this time including nearly equal numbers of females and males, with their symptom profiles matched as closely as possible.[20] Their data showed *increased* DMN connectivity in autistic females, as opposed to the underconnectivity showed by the mainly male cohorts in the 2017 survey, and greater connectivity to other frontal control systems. So, firm assertions with respect to characteristic underconnectivity in the autistic brain are not supported if you look at *all* autistic brains.

Where does this leave us in our quest to get autistic girls the recognition they need? Neuroscientists are waking up to the gaps in their models of the autistic brain and need to find a way to make them more representative of the whole autistic spectrum. Perhaps they should look more closely at camouflaging as a measure of what they have been missing?

KANNER-CHAMELEON DIFFERENCES IN THE AUTISTIC BRAIN: COULD CAMOUFLAGING HOLD THE KEY?

Camouflaging encapsulates key aspects of social behaviour. The close attention to social cues, and the production and rehearsal of social scripts, reflects a high-level quest to find out how to be socially successful. Additionally, camouflaging behaviour as a coping strategy reflects many of the regulated actions involved in being social, such as mimicking gestures or purposefully maintaining eye contact, or consciously suppressing autistic-like behaviours like stimming. You might recall one of my interviewees from chapter 4, who described living her daily life as being like an undercover agent, constantly monitoring her behaviour to check she didn't show up as an outsider.

This experience is echoed in so many of the personal testimonies of camouflaging autistic females, all speaking of a life on high alert. Their camouflaging is a survival mechanism, focussing fiercely on not being discovered as different, putting on their best normal to belong. Both qualitative and quantitative data indicate that a desire to fit in, to avoid the stigma of autism, is the main driving force behind camouflaging behaviour. Perhaps more than anything, the persistence of camouflaging behaviour, despite its association with high levels of mental health problems in autistic individuals, especially females, establishes a powerful motivational force behind social decisions that are superficially effective, but ultimately maladaptive.

Camouflaging in autism, therefore, could prove to be a useful index of atypical social processing at the level of both brain and behaviour. Particularly given the accumulating (if still biased) evidence of abnormalities in the social reward circuits in the autistic brain, camouflaging could be a fruitful focus for future research. As camouflaging is a pattern of autistic behaviour that, on average, is more common in females than males, targeting imaging studies on social reward circuits in the context of camouflaging behaviour could advance the understanding of sex/gender differences in autism.

A study by Meng-Chuan Lai and colleagues in 2019 examined sex and autism differences in parts of the theory-of-mind network, the brain bases of understanding others.[21] They used the self-monitoring (bony knees) task that we have come across before, where you are asked to think about yourself by pondering the question, 'How likely are you to think that keeping a diary is important?', or to think about what other people might be like by musing, for example, 'How likely is the queen/Harry Potter/your best friend to think that keeping a diary is important?' This kind of task should show some back and forth activity between the self-monitoring prefrontal areas of the brain and the other-monitoring areas, such as the temporoparietal junction.

The autistic males showed what is turning out to be predictably lower levels of activation in these areas than their neurotypical male peers. The autistic females, on the other hand, showed similar, if not slightly higher, levels of activation than typically developing females, and certainly higher than autistic males.

The researchers also measured camouflaging behaviour in their autistic participants and discovered that female levels were much higher. Intriguingly, the researchers showed that the higher the levels of camouflaging behaviour, the greater the levels of activation in those self-monitoring prefrontal areas. So the self–other monitoring pathways in the female autistic brain seem to be working on a par with typically developing females, although it does look as if there might be a tendency to an overactive self-checking system – completely on a par with being an undercover spy! Or as the authors put it: 'Autistic women may engage substantial insight about their own behaviours in interpersonal and social contexts – specifically, how their behaviours impact others, gauging and managing the impressions they make on others, updating the differences between their natural and camouflaged behaviours, and how such behaviours will achieve the desired goal of being perceived as neurotypical'.[22] Another example of autistic females prioritizing the avoidance of negative social experiences.

Another US team specifically focussed on the relationship between brain connectivity patterns and autistic camouflaging behaviour.[23] They found higher levels of camouflaging in autistic females, and this was associated with higher levels of connectivity in the brain's reward pathways, including the anterior cingulate and the striatum. The 'men-only' studies we looked at previously reported these areas as underconnected. This is another piece of evidence that a focus on the relationship between camouflaging behaviour and patterns of connectivity in reward pathways could offer a fruitful way forward in unpacking sex differences in the complex, multilevel associations between brain and behaviour in autism.

It is becoming clear that distinctive connectivity profiles could differentiate Kanner-like ASD individuals from chameleon-like ones. How does this evidence of different wiring patterns in the autistic brain fit into emerging ideas of brain function and social behaviour?

If you read the testimonies of camouflaging autistic females, so much of their anxieties concern the anticipation of what *might* go wrong. My family (and probably all families) is divided into two types. First, the 'what-ifs', who, on confronting just about any proposed activity, will instantly produce a list of difficulties that might be encountered: potentially cancelled trains, extreme weather events, or technological disasters. They will arrive at airports eight hours in advance of departure time 'just in case'; they will haul around suitcases packed with outfits to suit all eventualities from an August snowfall in Miami to a December heatwave in Iceland. In contrast, the 'whatever' members are last-minute planners and packers, blissfully unaware of the earthquake/tornado/blizzard probabilities in the country they are heading for, cheerily assuming there will be shops in their destination, so do not repeatedly double- or triple-check that they have remembered their phone charger/suncream/fur-lined gloves. They will arrive at train stations and airports with minutes to spare. Many of the autistic females I spoke to firmly identified themselves with my 'what-if' relatives, and said this exactly encapsulated their reasons for camouflaging. Every social encounter would be a what-if event and all their energies would be focussed on diverting social disaster.

This pattern is neatly summed up by Kate, one of my late-diagnosed interviewees, who had struggled with what was diagnosed as 'school phobia' in her primary school and then 'social anxiety' at her secondary school. She was diagnosed with autism in her thirties, when the psychologist who had just diagnosed her six-year-old daughter as autistic suggested that Kate displayed many of the same signs of autism:

> There are some days when I can't get out of bed because I am trapped by what-ifs. I wake up with my heart pounding – I'm already too anxious to think straight. My brain is locked in some kind of doom loop. I know I've got to do a presentation to my team. I have written and rewritten it and practised it to death – but what if someone asks a question I can't answer, what if the technology doesn't work, what if I get trapped in the lift on my way to the venue . . . what if the bloody sky falls in. I know that if I stay in bed, then none of the what-ifs will happen – so I stay in bed and the what-ifs win. I have no such thing as a mental shrug, or an 'I'll wing it' plan B. I wish there was a 'whatever' mode.

We are still in the early stages of studying the predictive coding process in autistic brains. The Zap the Aliens task, detailed in the previous chapter, allowed us to find a way of 'watching' how the brain generated a prediction when presented with repeated presentations of low-level sensory stimuli, and of showing that this process did not run as efficiently in autistic brains. Other groups have taken a slightly different approach and focussed on more social-type tasks, such as facial processing or emotion recognition.[24] You can show someone a very blurred image of a face and tell them that the face is expressing an emotion such as fear or happiness. Then you gradually reduce the blurriness and ask them to make a guess (via a button press) as soon as they think an emotion is recognizable. This means you can track how the brain gradually builds up a 'prior' ('I think it might be a happy face') until it makes a guess and a button press is generated. Accurate face-processing and emotion recognition are key features of social behaviour, so any difficulties could certainly undermine successful social interaction.

A study published in 2024 used this technique with autistic adults, both female and male, and matched controls.[25] What they found was intriguing. They were able to demonstrate that there are two key time windows in the path to identifying the stimulus. They equated the early stage, at about two hundred milliseconds, with the recognition that the image was a face, and the secondary stage, at about four hundred milliseconds, with the recognition of the emotion. In the first stage, autistic males showed reduced activation, suggesting general difficulties with face-processing. The brain activity of autistic females, on the other hand, was equivalent to that of the neurotypical groups. However, in the second time window, this autistic sex difference disappeared, and both females and males showed signs of slower processing. One way of interpreting this data is that autistic females do have some preserved, socially relevant, automatic skills – early stages of face-processing are intact – but the later, more complex skills – recognizing facially expressed emotion – are impaired. Which could fit in with the more detailed profile we now have of social abilities in autistic females. This might feel like a giant leap from how people deal with blurry faces – and this is just a single study, one of the first to take this kind of approach to the study of sex differences in autistic brains – but it could be a useful piece of the autism jigsaw.

AUTISM, SEX, AND THE SOCIAL WORLD

Twenty-first-century research into autism is bringing some long-needed changes into our understanding of this condition. We have a more nuanced understanding of the various stages of typical social behaviour, so it is possible to get a more detailed picture of where autistic individuals have difficulties, and why most autistic individuals find the social world such an obstacle course.

Understanding other people or decoding a social situation will involve several stages. The first and simplest one is based on what you can see or hear – this could be facial expression, body language, gestures, tone of voice, the available cues that we might focus on in order to work out what is going on, where we fit in, what we might need to do next. Research and personal reports show that autistic individuals can struggle even at this level. Then there are the 'invisibles' – the mind-reading skills that help you understand the mental states of the person or people you are trying to relate to – does that tone of voice or facial expression mean they really want to make you welcome, or are they actually obeying some external social rules of politeness that you haven't grasped? How do you establish a 'social prior' if you don't seem to have access to the necessary rules? We already know that this kind of mind-reading can be problematic if you are on the spectrum. Camilla Pang, an autistic scientist, captures this puzzlement in the opening lines of her award-winning book, *Explaining Humans*: 'It was five years into my life on Earth that I started to think I'd landed in the wrong place. I must have missed the stop. I felt like a stranger within my own species: someone who understood the words but couldn't speak the language'.[26]

And you may remember Rachel, from chapter 4, who described the invisibility of social rules as akin to the difficulties that deaf people have in understanding the exchange of sound between hearing people having conversations.

These are powerful testimonies not only to the short-sightedness of the blanket assumption that autistic individuals are lacking in social motivation, but also to the astonishing insights that autistic individuals have into their own difficulties. They also reveal how much more of an understanding of autism (and, indeed the social world) you get if you actually talk to autistic people! We are starting to get clues as to why autistic females might have different difficulties with the social world than autistic males. The brain research community is starting to wake up to the rather scandalous evidence that females have been missing from decades of autism research and, again, uncovering evidence that the brain bases of autism might be different for females.

There is another arena in which issues of sex and gender and autism play out in complex ways, and that is in the world of adolescence. The fragile compensatory systems may crumble; camouflaging no longer offers a carefully constructed invisibility cloak; the social world becomes more complex, more demanding, and quite possibly more cruel. This appears to impact autistic females more profoundly; indeed, it may be the first time that the possibility they are autistic is even raised. And an autism diagnosis may be entangled with other behavioural problems such as eating disorders and self-harm.

Adolescence is a time when socialization pressures, especially gendered expectations, exert powerful influences. It is also a time when dramatic brain changes are occurring, almost invariably more problematic in brains that are not typically wired. It is to this pivotal stage of life that we now turn.

CHAPTER 8

FEMALE, AUTISTIC, AND ADOLESCENT

THE PERFECT STORM?

We now have an emerging awareness of the presence of a significant group of 'differently different' autistic individuals, the majority of whom are female, who appear to be highly focussed on social engagement, but share the fundamental autistic difficulties with their internal social navigation system. Imagine, then, how this group could be affected by the trials and tribulations of adolescence. Adolescence is a time of massive physical and social change. And bear in mind that a highly significant and often overlooked characteristic of nearly all autistic individuals is a powerful aversion to change. It is a time when all brains, autistic and non-autistic, are undergoing phases of dramatic reorganization; when all bodies are being altered by powerful waves of hormonally induced changes. In many societies, adolescence may also mark a relocation to a new and potentially hostile environment – a new school – when old friends and new peers seem to be acquiring novel and different identities. On top of all this there is the constant formation and reformation of 'friendship' groupings, cliques and baffling alliances, based on mysterious membership rules, combined with powerful pressures to conform or be excluded.

It can be an ugly time. The statistics on 'peer victimization' (or bullying) are stark. In the UK, a 2023 report from the Department for Education revealed that 40 per cent of fourteen- to fifteen-year-olds reported being bullied in the preceding twelve months. In the US in 2021, about 20 per cent of students aged twelve to eighteen report being bullied. A 2022 survey revealed online bullying to be a major problem for more than half (53 per cent) of US teens. It is a worldwide problem: UNESCO reports overall rates of about 30 per cent.[1] Adolescents with ASD are victimized and bullied at exceptionally high rates (46–94 per cent), much more frequently than neurotypical youth (10–15 per cent) and other disability groups.[2] It also appears there are gender differences in these bullying activities. ASD boys are much more likely to be physically bullied or socially ignored, whereas girls are more likely to be victims of 'relational aggression', such as spreading rumours, gossiping, and/or ostracism. Given that autistic girls are particularly driven by the need to belong, this kind of social rejection will have an exceptionally powerful impact.

It is clearly also a mentally troubling time. The World Health Organization estimates that, worldwide, one in seven ten- to nineteen-year-olds experience mental health problems. A survey published by the UK National Health Service in 2020 showed that one in six young people (aged five to sixteen) experienced some kind of mental health problem in 2020 (up from one in nine in 2017). In 2023 this number had risen again to one in five. In the US, a CDC survey in 2021 reported that 29 per cent of high school students experienced poor mental health. In 2023, a further report showed that this problem was significantly greater for adolescent girls, with twice as many visits to emergency departments for mental health issues than for adolescent boys, and suspected suicide attempts four times higher among teenage girls than boys.[3]

The statistics are even more grim for autistic adolescents.[4] Anxiety and depression are a particular problem. The incidence of diagnosable anxiety disorders is approximately 60 per cent greater in this group than neurotypicals, and a fourfold increase in depressive disorders has been reported.[5] The statistics for autistic female adolescents are even worse, with reports of 35.3 per cent diagnosed with depression as opposed to 9.4 per cent of non-autistic females. Mental health problems that commonly emerge in adolescence, such as eating disorders and self-harm, are also much more common in autistic adolescent females.[6]

Psychologists Giorgia Picci and Suzanne Scherf have proposed a two-hit model of autism, with the first hit caused by disrupted neural development, setting up a neural system 'built to fail', and the second hit linked to a combination of neural re-organization and hormonal changes in adolescence, in concert with the increasing complexity of the social environment.[7] Their 2015 review paper on this model marshals some powerful data to support this approach; sex/gender differences do not even get a mention. This is perhaps forgivable as we know that little detailed attention had been paid to females on the spectrum prior to 2015. But the proposal provides a useful framework for us to investigate if and why adolescence is such a problematic time for autistic females.

DOES ADOLESCENCE IMPACT AUTISTIC FEMALES DIFFERENTLY?

For many of our differently different group, it was not until these turbulent times of adolescence that their autism was even recognized. It is clear from personal testimonies (especially from late-diagnosed women) that there are a large number of young, pre-teenage people who have suffered in silence, or flown beneath the diagnostic radar, during their primary school years and remained unidentified. This information fitted in with the existing narrative that autism was a male problem, with many of these invisible autists being girls.

One point worth remembering is that autism is considered a lifelong developmental disorder, present from birth (or before), and normally diagnosed within the first three or four years of life (or earlier when the presenting problems are more marked). So you would not expect to see age-related increases in prevalence. A UK-based study in 2020 looked at the timing of autism diagnosis in a cohort of 581 children.[8] It found that, although over 70 per cent of the children were diagnosed in primary school, this left nearly 30 per cent who were not diagnosed until secondary school (despite parental and/or teacher concerns about social difficulties in this group being raised at or before the age of five years in 75 per cent of this group). What was behind this delay in diagnosis? As well as factors including degree of intellectual impairment or symptom severity, and low household income and neighbourhood health deprivation, another determining factor was whether the child was female or male, with more girls than boys not receiving an autism diagnosis until secondary school.

A team tracking the development of autistic social traits in a large UK-based birth cohort study, using the Social Communication Disorder Scale, studied sex differences in 4,960 females and 4,784 males at ages seven, ten, thirteen, and sixteen years.[9]

The picture they found showed that boys, on average, had higher levels of autistic social traits at age seven, which declined slightly and then showed a small increase between ten and sixteen. Girls, on the other hand, showed a different pattern of change. Starting off lower than boys, they showed a marked escalation of autistic social traits from the age of ten. By the age of sixteen they had equivalent, if not marginally higher, levels of autistic traits than boys.

The researchers also explored those children who scored above the clinical threshold on the checklist, that is, who should actually be diagnosed as autistic. There were higher numbers of boys at age seven (10 per cent of the total) as compared to girls (5 per cent of the total) but by age sixteen this difference had disappeared, with those passing the clinical threshold comprising 8.6 per cent of the boys and 9.3 per cent of the girls.

So the evidence shows that the kind of social difficulties that will 'earn' an autistic diagnosis only become apparent in some autistic females during adolescence. There are a few potential explanations for this phenomenon.

One model, an extension of the two-hit proposition mentioned above, invokes some kind of thresholding effect, where the onset of puberty has disrupted or deactivated biological or behavioural protective mechanisms that have, to that point, either prevented the presentation of autism, or disguised its presence.[10] Perhaps a brain that is already functioning at reduced capacity because of disordered connectivity development is overwhelmed by the demands of adolescent brain reorganization. During adolescence, the brain's cognitive control centres and emotional processing centres are temporarily disconnected. In autism, we know the emotional processing centres can be overactive from birth. In some autistic individuals, cognitive processing can equally be a challenge. So we have an already precariously balanced network going temporarily offline and at the same time having to deal with the much greater personal and social challenges that come with adolescence.

In other words, the painstakingly constructed scaffolding of compensatory or camouflaging strategies is no longer fit for purpose. Life as an adolescent has become much, much more complicated, peer pressure to conform and fit in is overwhelming, and the bewildered autistic adolescent can be confronted with increasingly sophisticated ways of being socially rejected and ostracized, against which they have little defence. This layered threat is captured by Laura James in her book *Odd Girl Out*, writing about the isolation she experienced at school:

> The girls at school seemed to have a secret briefing that informed them of exactly how to behave. When they huddled together in the playground, the conversations bounced without missing a beat from boys to cherry mint lip gloss . . . . They touched each other easily, too, applying mascara to each other's lashes . . . linking arms as they walked across the playground. . . . I wanted so much to be part of that and, although I did sometimes get invited along, I was never quite in the middle of the group. I was always on the edge, always getting it slightly wrong, never quite feeling part of things.[11]

In addition, there is the greater occurrence in autistic females of a range of disturbing (and possibly disabling) adolescent mental health conditions that, in themselves, may overshadow or distract from the underlying autistic condition. Ironically, this is where we can hit what looks like *female* spotlight problem. Eating disorders, for example, have been firmly established as a female problem, so if an adolescent female (who may well be an undiagnosed autist) presents with a life-threatening pattern of disordered eating, the default diagnosis – and her treatment – will focus on her eating problem.[12] Here we have the issue of whether what looks like an eating problem is actually a manifestation of autism, whether the autism renders autistic females more vulnerable to eating disorders, or whether there is a genuine co-occurrence of autism and certain mental health problems.

Perhaps the particular cocktail of genetic variation that can produce autism could also produce other patterns of atypical behaviour as well.[13] Whether or not their autism was also evident, the behavioural presentation should be ticking all the right boxes for their 'other' problems. If not, then it is more likely that we are looking at a misdiagnosis, and spotting where the differences lie may well provide some more insights into autism. The timing of this 'sudden' emergence of difficulties in girls could well be telling too.

Direct evidence about the sources of these greater difficulties in autistic adolescent females is, as ever, hard to come by. We shall have to step back and see what we can learn by comparisons between typical and autistic teenage brains and behaviour, and then dig deeper to see if we can extract anything specific to being female.

THE TYPICAL TEENAGE BRAIN

We used to think that the teenage brain was just a not-quite-grown-up brain, a bit bigger than an infant's, a bit smaller than an adult's, the various structures gradually reaching full size, the pathways between them gradually developing. It was known that there was an ongoing programme of 'pruning' and reorganization, with the stunning nerve cell growth that happens in the early years of brain development followed by a process of elimination' of nerve cells and tidying-up of nerve cell connections. The metaphor of training rambling roses is much used, but highly accurate. It was assumed this programme ran steadily, from baby brain to the full-grown version, with no marked variation along the way.

But, until relatively recently, we didn't have direct access to this ongoing landscaping of the brain, being mainly reliant on autopsies or animal studies. It was the advent of human brain-imaging techniques at the end of the last century that meant that such changes could be viewed over time in the same (living) brains. As we know from earlier chapters, it is now possible, for example, to track changes in grey matter (nerve cell bodies) and white matter (connecting pathways). We can also see the creation and activation of different networks carrying out different functions, from responding to simple sensory changes to solving complex social problems, such as identifying members of a social gathering as in-group or out-group, and deciding what kind of social script needs to be selected accordingly.

We also know there is a set of structures that control all aspects of social behaviour. This can include the development of a sense of our own self and the storage of social scripts, embedded in the activities of our prefrontal cortex. Our attempts at understanding other people, involving the anticipation of their intentions, likes, and dislikes, draw on the interaction between our temporal lobe–based memories of other people and events, and our parietal lobe–based perceptions and interpretations of social situations. We have also identified a social GPS navigation system, centred around the ACC, that regulates our social behaviour, encouraging anything that will reinforce group membership, and discouraging anything that could lead to social rejection or ostracism.

This response control centre is linked to activation in core components of the emotional processing system – the amygdala, the insula, and the striatum. This connection ensures that our social behaviour is appropriately tagged with, for example, the joy of the right response admitting us to our in-group or the despair of the wrong move leading to social rejection.

Once we were able to identify these key elements and also link them to longitudinal studies of developing brains, it became clear that the trajectory of brain growth does not comprise a nice smooth journey from baby brain to adult brain. There is a very specific time of really intense brain re-landscaping that coincides with puberty and the teenage years. And a major area of restructuring seems to involve the social brain.

One of the first reports of adolescent-specific brain changes was from a small-scale longitudinal study of children aged four to twenty-two years, who had been scanned every two years.[14] The report showed that there was a dramatic period of grey matter changes around the time of puberty. Grey matter had increased until this time window and then quite sharply declined, with the rates of decline varying across different parts of the brain. White matter showed a different pattern, increasing steadily throughout puberty until the early twenties. So it is not only the bodies of teenagers that change with puberty; their brains do too.

A UK-based consortium of brain-imaging labs gathered data from over two thousand participants over three time points between the ages of fourteen and twenty-two to examine how brain networks and the connections between them changed at these various stages.[15] The overall picture was that the strength of short-range connections decreased as the brain matured – indicating established efficiency in basic sensory and motor control – but the strength of long-range connections increased –

paralleling the development of more complex information processing functions. Using such measures of connectivity, it quickly became clear that changes in the teenage brain were not just a simple tidying-up business; there was a lot of rerouting going on.

The researchers found two distinct patterns of changes in brain connectivity. The 'conservative' changes were in well-established pathways linked to sensory processing; these just got stronger (the 'rich get richer' effect). The 'disruptive' changes were between the higher-level information processing parts of the cortex (especially those linked to social cognition, including the understanding of other people). In some cases, relatively strong connections were dismantled; in others weaker ones were strengthened. There will be phases where previously established pathways, for instance between emotion-regulation and frontal regulatory areas, will be in the process of being dismantled, and newer control systems not yet established. These can be linked to the teenage behaviour we all know too well.

TYPICAL TEENAGE BRAINS AND TYPICAL TEENAGE BEHAVIOUR

You don't have to be a neuroscientist to know that adolescents' behaviour can be as turbulent as their brain changes might lead us to expect. An emerging sense of self (and self needs!), a frantic need for peer approval, dramatic emotional outbursts, and apparent lack of any impulse control will be familiar scenarios in most families. All of these processes, as we know from looking at the social brain in adults, are core features of the activities of the social brain, and can be modelled for investigation in the scanner.

With respect to issues of identity, developmental psychologists have shown the onset of puberty is associated with the emergence of self-consciousness or self-awareness.

Looking at brain imagers' use of the kind of self-referencing tasks that we met in chapter 6 (yes, it is bony elbows again), we know that parts of the prefrontal cortex become activated when we are processing information about ourselves. Similarly, activation of the so-called default mode network, when we are theoretically doing nothing but actually indulging in a lot of self-centred daydreaming, has been shown to be a strong index of a focus on the self. You may not be surprised to learn that there are significantly higher levels of activity in these parts of the brain in adolescent participants.[16] A lot of self-focussed daydreaming going on perhaps!

Another measure of the emerging self-concept involves what is called the 'looking-glass self', which is the idea that a lot of self-reference involves what other people think of you.[17] Additions to the list of self-referencing questions might be 'Would you agree with the statement, "People think I am shy"?' Such a question conjures the idea of the imaginary audience, a common adolescent notion that others are judgementally sizing you up. During this task, higher levels of activation were again recorded in the adolescent prefrontal cortex. So not only do you think a lot about yourself when you are an adolescent, you are powerfully concerned about how other people view this self.

Difficulties with response inhibition and emotion regulation have been investigated using a go/no-go task. Participants were told to press a button if they were shown a picture of an emotionless or neutral face, but NOT to respond if the image of a face showed an emotion ('Don't respond to the smiley face').[18] Typical adolescents were appallingly bad at this, and showed many more 'false alarms' (pressing the button when the face DID express an emotion) than either adults or, importantly, younger children. Adolescents also showed much higher levels of activation in the ventral striatum, part of the emotion regulation and reward system in the social brain. This heightened responsiveness to reward could underpin the adventure-seeking and risk-taking behaviours characteristic of adolescents. We now know that many brain changes associated with adolescence start at the back of the brain, and happen before changes involving frontal areas. This means that there will be stages when parts of a network will 'mature' before others. In more advanced forms of human behaviour, control systems are commonly arranged in a top-down fashion, so what has been characterized as a lack of 'self-control' in adolescents could, in brain terms, be exactly that, reflecting the potency of a freshly upgraded reward system not yet fitted with its prefrontal speed limiter.

The consequences of this imbalance between a cautious cognitive monitoring system and an unharnessed emotional system were neatly demonstrated in a study that had children, adolescents, and adults playing a gambling version of a go/no-go task. Monetary rewards and punishments were linked to high- and low-stakes clues, warning you that, in the high-stakes condition, for example, you could win $1.00 as opposed to $0.20 if you were right, but lose $0.50 as opposed to $0.10 if you were wrong.[19] In this kind of task, you would expect to see improved performance with the higher-stakes version, demonstrating a recognition of the value of performing the task correctly. Here, only the older participants (nineteen to twenty years old) showed this improvement. The difference in the stakes did not affect the performance of the younger players, who were less efficient at the task whether the stakes were high or low. At the brain level, the defining characteristic of the better performers (besides their age) was increased recruitment of the prefrontal areas and, perhaps crucially, more powerful connections between the prefrontal cortex and the reward centres of the brain.

Effectively, this study demonstrated the emerging efficiency of a 'cool' cognitive control system moderating a 'hot' motivational assessment system, resulting in the appropriate balance between the rewards offered and the actions required to maximize performance. If your brain is younger, you are not very good at matching what you need to do with what you will gain if you get it right, or lose if you get it wrong. What we are looking at here is evidence of an adolescent lack of the necessary fine-tuning in the reward system. Anyone who has ever sat down with an adolescent to get them to engage with future-focussed decision-making, such as filling in higher education application forms or making career choices, will be familiar with the power of short-term gains in the teenage brain.

Another aspect of adolescence is the powerful (sometimes all-conquering) effect of peer pressure. Again, cognitive neuroscience can help us get a handle on what is going on. One part of the system's reorganization in the adolescent brain involves improving the connections within, but more importantly between, different components of the newly remodelled cortical networks. One revealing study was carried out by Marie-Hélène Grosbras and colleagues from the Brain and Body Centre at the University of Nottingham.[20] They compared brain activation patterns in adolescents who scored high or low on a measure of resistance to peer influence. Participants had to indicate which of a pair of statements about social interactions was most true of themselves. For example, 'Some people hide their true opinion from their friends if they think their friends will make fun of them because of it', and, 'Other people will say their true opinion in front of their friends, even if they know their friends will make fun of them because of it'. Responses generated a low or high score indicating individuals' resistance to peer pressure.

Then, in the MRI scanner, the participants watched video clips of either neutral or negative stimuli such as impassive or angry faces. The fMRI data showed that individuals with less resistance to peer influence showed much greater levels of brain reactivity when presented with negative social stimuli, consistent with a much more powerful emotional response to such information. Those resistant to peer influence showed greater co-ordination between the prefrontal cortex and social regulatory systems, a measure of a more controlled and less over-emotional response. These results suggest that individuals most likely to respond to peer pressure are more reactive to negative social stimuli, and that the lower connectivity with regulatory systems may result in a greater lack of control over associated responses. Admittedly, this was a small-scale correlational study, but its results are consistent with emerging models of the importance of network co-ordination in maturing brains.

Another study involved nine- to seventeen-year-olds in a pretend chat room session.[21] While the children were in the scanner, they were asked to rate how interested they were in their chat room peers, and then to think how these peers might rate them. In females, but not the males, there was an increasing activation, with age, in brain areas involved with emotion regulation and salience processing, including the insula. This ties in with other evidence that adolescent females show greater concern about peer evaluation and respond more powerfully to social stimuli.

A useful measure of the importance of peer influence is how your self-esteem is impacted by rejection or criticism from friends and significant others. Behavioural studies have shown that adolescents show much higher levels of anxiety in such situations than adults. Again, there are quite marked sex differences here, with girls appearing to attach much more significance to peer evaluation than boys.[22]

How is this social rejection experience reflected in the brain? As we have seen, there are a range of mischievous manipulations that cognitive neuroscientists have dreamed up to model social rejection experiences in the scanner. One of the most popular is the Cyberball game.[23] In this video game, participants can see themselves depicted as a cartoon character, enjoying a game of catch with two other players. Eventually, these two players start excluding the participant and only pass the ball between themselves, the peer exclusion condition. At the beginning and end of each scanning session, participants are asked to rate their levels of self-esteem. Similarly, after being excluded they are asked to report their levels of distress. This study reveals the balance between the self-monitoring and social control processes linked to activity in the prefrontal cortex, and the distress responses, shown by activity in the emotional coding systems (linked to the insula). The greater the distress, the lower the prefrontal responses and the higher the insula responses. Activation in the behavioural regulatory system centred on the anterior cingulate will also be triggered. In the absence of the calming influence of the prefrontal cortex, the behavioural consequences of the punctured self-esteem caused by social rejection (even when it is only by a cartoon character in a video game) are almost invariably emotional withdrawal, self-criticism, and lack of further engagement – also known as going off in a huff and slamming the door, perhaps.

A team from UCLA compared brain responses in adolescents and adults using the Cyberball game and found some intriguing differences.[24] Adults showed interacting patterns of activity in all parts of the social brain network – some prefrontal self-monitoring activity, a certain amount of regulatory control ('keep calm and carry on'), and the occasional flash of insula activity ('huh'). So, yes, it looked like they found the game an emotionally distressing, negative experience, but the normal brain checks and balances were in place – 'I'm miffed that I'm being left out of this game, but I must remember that it is only a game'. The adolescents were more fired up – some prefrontal self-monitoring activity similar to adults ('How come I'm not being included?'), but less regulatory control ('I'll keep pressing the button till they let me join in') and a fully fired-up emotional processing centre ('What the hell?!'). The greater their reported distress, the greater the insula activity. Cue yet another game controller being smashed against the wall!

A SADLY REAL-LIFE FORM OF SOCIAL REJECTION IS BULLYING, doubly impactful in adolescence given the importance of peer relations. Does the experience of being bullied affect how you respond to social rejection? A brain-imaging study from Germany, again using the Cyberball task, investigated this and showed that the amount of bullying teenagers experienced appeared to affect their response to social rejection.[25] Those who reported the most bullying experiences showed the strongest increase in activation in the predicted social brain areas, including the prefrontal cortex and the anterior cingulate. The brains of bullied adolescents seemed to magnify the Cyberball effect. Higher levels of self-referencing and plummeting self-esteem ('This really matters, they all hate me') linked to a pattern of maladaptive behavioural response such as inhibition and withdrawal or self-silencing.

The typically developing teenage brain, then, is characterized by a programme of quite dramatic re-organization of its connectivity, with associated changes in behaviour. The drama of peer evaluation and social rejection plays out more powerfully in the adolescent brain.

What happens in the autistic brain? We already know that the autistic brain, from infancy onwards, is characterized by anomalous connections, both within and between brain networks. It is highly probable, then, that adolescence-based brain changes in these very connections will cause yet further disruption, with the emergence of different behavioural difficulties.

THE AUTISTIC TEENAGE BRAIN

Early models of the developing autistic brain suggested that it is characterized by hyperconnectivity, linked to exuberant cell growth, particularly within specialized brain networks. However, studies of autistic adults more commonly reported evidence of reduced connectivity. This suggests that at some stage, there might be some form of overcorrection in autistic brain connectivity patterns. Given what we now know about brain development in typical brains, it is probable that this overcorrection could occur during adolescence, with an excess of the normal cellular pruning processes.

A key study on the subject is by Katherine Lawrence and colleagues from UCLA.[26] This was a longitudinal study, with connectivity measures taken in the same group of typically developing and autistic participants within a three-year time period (at twelve years old and fifteen years old approximately). They examined connectivity between three of the main networks in the social brain – the default mode (or self-referencing, daydreaming) network, the social reward (or salience) network, and the regulatory, decision-making network that is based in the prefrontal cortex, linked to the ACC. These have been shown to be strongly interconnected in non-autistic adults, with patterns of activation between the various components varying dependent on task demands.

In typically developing adolescents, there was a pattern of gradually reducing connectivity between these three networks, suggesting a move away from the all-or-none type response of younger years. Patterns of measured activation were showing a more on-off relationship between the networks. When one was active the others were less so, suggesting a more balanced use of brain resources. In autistic individuals, there was much less evidence of reducing connectivity, and the interplay between the various networks was much less measured. In some cases, high levels of activity in the default mode network suggested a constantly active self-referencing system, perhaps overpowering a behavioural control system, with a volatile reward system thrown into the mix. If you were wondering if this is true of both females and males, in the autistic group, there were sixteen participants, only one of whom was female. In the control group, all twenty-two participants were male. An interesting insight then, but once again, only part of the story.

How about the effects of social rejection in autistic adolescents, given that this was an area where typically developing adolescents showed a specific pattern of responses different from adults? This study has been followed up with a group of autistic participants by the same neuroimaging centre at UCLA, once again using the Cyberball task.[27] Both typical and autistic groups of adolescents reported the same moderate levels of distress after the game. However, the autistic group showed much lower levels of brain activation in the anterior cingulate and the insula, which might suggest that, although the autistic participants were aware that being left out of an online game was not a great social experience, their brains were not coding the event as some kind of significant, brain-altering experience – the brain's equivalent of a 'whatever' shrug.

This report of reduced brain activation during socially important events is consistent with previous reports in the adult autistic population. But, of course, we only know that such hypo-activation was true of males on the spectrum, as females weren't generally being included in such studies. When female autistic participants were included, in other studies looking at social reward processing, on average they had *higher* levels of brain activity. Could we find out if such differences were also true of adolescents by looking at the results of the above study? No, because, of the nineteen autistic participants, eighteen were male.

Fortunately, as we saw in the previous chapter, we can get an inkling as to how brain responses in adolescent autistic females might be different from those of adolescent autistic males by looking at studies using participants recruited from the GENDAAR cohort, specifically focussing on autistic female-male comparisons. If you recall, one such study found that autistic girls displayed *increased* activity during social rewards, compared to autistic boys.[28] The autistic girls also showed greater reactivity in the anterior insula compared to typically developing girls. Little sign of the 'whatever' shrug here, then.

Evidence, then, suggests that the development of the brain in adolescence is different for autistic individuals. Poorly established brain connectivity patterns are further disrupted, and increased difficulties with peer interactions appear to affect the reactivity in social brain networks. The evidence of whether or not this plays out differently in females and males is frustratingly limited, but a pattern is emerging. It appears that there is increased reactivity in self-referencing and social coding networks in females as opposed to under-reactivity in males. This could well underpin behavioural observations that autistic-like behaviour becomes more apparent in females during adolescence, to the extent that previously undiagnosed individuals may cross the clinical threshold. So the effects of changes in their adolescent brains has undermined the previously hard-won protective camouflage that kept these girls under the radar during their primary school years.

In addition, as we have noted, adolescence is a time of increasing mental health problems in non-autistic populations, but rates are much higher in autistic ones. There are reports of prevalence rates of 70 to 90 per cent of autistic adolescents having at least one co-occurring psychiatric disorder. Here at least there is a well-developed evidence base on sex differences. Mood disorders and anxiety disorders are reportedly more prevalent in females, whereas attention deficit hyperactivity disorder (ADHD), schizophrenia, and obsessive-compulsive disorder are more prevalent in males.[29]

There are particular adolescent mental health problems that are more common in females, where a considerable overlap between the core characteristics of the condition and aspects of both the female autism phenotype and the female autism experience has been noted. For example, heightened anxiety about social group membership and atypical responsiveness to negative social experiences is more common in autistic females. They also suffer more from bullying and abuse. These have been identified as key factors in cases of self-harming, or non-suicidal self-injury (NSSI). There can also be close associations between the symptom profiles of certain eating disorders and of female autism, such as rigid routines around food choice, or obsessive aversion to change. Are such conditions unfortunately co-occurring in unusually high percentages in autistic women, or is there some kind of entangled causal relationship between them? Or are clinicians, faced with troubled girls ('who don't get autism') just reaching for alternatives from among the labels of things that girls do get?

We could think about these vulnerabilities in adolescent autistic females in the context of looking at *all* forms of mental illness to see if any kind of common pattern might emerge. For example, we have come across the notion that many psychopathological issues in females can be categorized as 'internalizing' problems, with women expressing their mental distresses by turning in on or 'attacking' themselves. Indeed, we have speculated that this might be behind the 'paler' appearance of autism in girls, as characterized by Sukhareva so many decades ago. Sarah Wild, the head teacher of Limpsfield Grange, the only state-funded residential school for girls with special needs in the UK, observes that when autistic girls suffer mental health problems they are much more likely to 'implode emotionally'.[30]

Internalizing distress can present as physically self-destructive behaviours such as eating disorders or self-harm, both of which are found at high levels in female autistic populations. Perhaps if we look at some of the research findings individually relevant to such conditions, as well as examining the common factors and areas of overlap, we might shed some more light on female autism.

FEMALE AUTISM AND EATING DISORDERS

There are several categories of clinically diagnosed eating disorders, including anorexia nervosa (AN), bulimia, and binge-eating disorder but, with respect to autism, the focus has mainly been on anorexia. AN is an eating disorder with peak onset in adolescence, between fifteen and nineteen years. It is significantly more common in females, with some estimates of 10:1 female:male ratios. The prevalence of AN in the general population has been estimated as about 4 per cent among females and 0.3 per cent in males.[31] There appears to be a high prevalence of autism among AN patients, and a high prevalence of AN in female eating disordered populations.[32] So adolescence is a time when a particular mental health issue rears its ugly head, and appears to strike autistic females harder than their neurotypical sisters.

Historically, there has been speculation that AN may even be a form of female autism, with some kind of common biological factor expressing itself differently in girls, who developed anorexia, as opposed to boys, who were autistic. In 1983, the psychiatrist Christopher Gillberg wrote a letter to the *British Journal of Psychiatry* reporting on three families where a boy with autism had close female relatives with AN, speculating that the two conditions might have a common source that presented differently in females and males:

> The obsessive insistence on sameness seen in autistic children is sometimes a striking phenomenon in anorexia nervosa too. Is there a possibility that a common biochemical disturbance may interact with other factors (brain damage, starvation, cultural factors) to cause autism in young boys and anorexia nervosa in prepubertal girls?[33]

Gillberg's letter led to suggestions that autism's missing girls might be found among the ranks of anorexia sufferers. It was reported that 20–35 per cent of girls and women with anorexia met the clinical criteria for autism.[34] Atypical eating behaviours are certainly common in autism – a 2019 study reported that 70 per cent of the autistic children they studied showed some form of unusual eating behaviour, often in the form of very limited food preferences or aversion to particular textures.[35] Given that there are anorexic girls who are not autistic and autistic girls who are not anorexic, the notion of the interchangeability of the two conditions was clearly an oversimplification. But attention to traits that indicated some kind of overlap was revealing.

One suggestion has been that what looks like autistic behaviour in anorexic populations is actually a consequence of chronic starvation, which can be associated with avoidance of social interactions, inflexibility and rigid insistence on routines, and lack of emotional responsivity, particularly in the face of the high levels of distress that eating disorders can cause for families and friends. But there is strong evidence that autistic traits preceded the onset of anorexia in many sufferers, and also that some weight-recovered anorexics continue to exhibit such traits.[36]

Those anorexic females who had an additional confirmed diagnosis of autism often presented with higher levels of eating disorder severity.[37] They were more likely to have extremely low body mass index, to have been tube-fed, and to have experienced a record number of purging episodes. So was autism some kind of primary cause of AN, more relentlessly driving it on than might be the case with the body image or weight concern issues more commonly expressed in anorexic girls without autism? I spoke about this to Sarah Wild. She suggested that the co-occurring incidence may be related to autistic girls' passionate need to fit into a (or any) community and that, in an eating disorder unit, these girls could well be slavishly copying the behaviours around them. She wryly commented that if an autistic girl was admitted to an anorexia clinic, characteristic levels of perfectionism could drive her to be the 'best' anorexic there was, copying each and every manifestation of the condition, and competing for the kudos attached to the need for more extreme interventions, such as intubation. In *Good Girls*, her memoir about her own experiences of anorexia, the journalist Hadley Freeman describes how you could acquire a 'cool' status in an eating disorders unit:

> Do you know what makes you cool on an eating disorders ward? . . . It's if you've been fed intravenously. It doesn't matter if you've had seventeen admissions and you're riddled with osteoporosis. If you haven't had the tube then you're just a day tripper.[38]

As we've noted before, matters of identity figure large in discussions of female autism, when a key benefit of an eventual diagnosis appears to be that of finally feeling that you know who you are and where you belong, a sense of finding your tribe. Which resonates with what Sarah Wild had to say. And, as it happens, the same issue crops up in discussions of anorexia, where resistance to treatment can be linked to a fear of the loss of a sense of self, which has become inextricably mixed with their anorexia – 'Who am I without my eating disorder?'[39] So identity and belongingness are powerful drivers of both anorexic behaviour and autism.

Such issues are evident in comments from autistic girls and women with anorexia reported in a report entitled '"For me, the anorexia is just a symptom, and the cause is the autism": Investigating restrictive eating disorders in autistic women'.[40] Here, sixteen women provide hugely thoughtful insights into their own experiences, for instance: 'I have never had much of a sense of self, and I think possibly [anorexia] then became a little bit like an identity. Going into hospital and being aware that everybody has the same condition, you then do become a lot more aware of some of the anorexia traits and you do sort of take them on'.

As ever, the voices of autistic women themselves offer the clearest insight into what might be driving their disordered eating. It is definitely not always about weight concern or body image, which appears to be the most powerful factor in anorexia, for example, and the target of many of the psychological therapies. In chapter 3, we mentioned Christine McGuiness's documentary *Unmasking My Autism*, a wide-ranging exploration of what she found it was like to be autistic.[41] She discussed her own history of eating disorders, and compared notes with Fi, another autistic woman who was struggling with an ongoing eating disorder. Both agreed that the reason they had restricted their food intake was primarily around sensory issues, such as the avoidance of certain smells and textures, limiting themselves to what was called 'the beige diet'. They admitted to being driven by inflexible rituals around eating, and by obsessions with calorie counting and exercise routines, or by beliefs about healthy or harmful eating. Again, these patterns of behaviour were not linked to weight control. Anorexia also seemed to offer them a form of escape from the unpredictable confusion of real life. As Fi observed in her conversation with Christine McGuiness: 'This anorexia came for me. It took me out of the world and put me into a world that I could understand. . . . And it gave me something that I felt I could get right'.[42]

There is a newly recognized form of eating disorder, and here the overlap with autistic behaviour is much more striking. Avoidant/restrictive food intake disorder (ARFID) was included in DSM for the first time in the latest version, DSM-5. ARFID is defined as an eating or feeding disorder characterized by a persistent and disturbed pattern of feeding or eating that leads to a failure to meet nutritional/energy needs.[43] Unusually for eating disorders, ARFID diagnoses have a fairly even female:male ratio, which might make it seem irrelevant when searching for clues about female autism. However, in discussions about ARFID, there are clear echoes of discussions about combined anorexia and autism in women. Its symptoms include a relative absence of concern about body image or weight gain, but a hyper-focus on avoiding certain types of food, due to sensory qualities such as texture or smell, or establishing very restrictive eating rituals. See 'the beige diet' described above! And the descriptions of autism-linked RRBIs are clearly being played out in such food intake obsessions.

Several of the autistic women I spoke to said they had to make sure that certain types of food didn't touch their plate – tackling a full English breakfast involved a sausage barrier to keep runny baked beans away from dried food, for example, or refusing to eat anything new, or red.

A study published in 2021 looked at genetic risk factors for ARFID in a large autism cohort.[44] Using a range of questions about any form of avoidant or restrictive food intake, it revealed that 21 per cent of the autistic group were at high risk of ARFID, as were up to 17 per cent of their parents. There was no evidence of females being more vulnerable than males, but those aspects of autism most closely linked to ARFID, particularly around rigid routines, insistence on sameness, and sensory sensitivities echo the female personal testimonies we have seen throughout the book.

On the surface, the presentation of eating disorders such as anorexia and the disordered eating behaviour linked to autism might seem to be so interchangeable you could easily pick the label you would more commonly associate with females. Interviews with those who have received both an eating disorder diagnosis and an autism diagnosis are telling (and familiar). In the paper mentioned previously describing the experiences of women with joint autism/eating disordered problems ('"For me, the anorexia is just a symptom, and the cause is the autism" . . .'), it's revealed that all sixteen women had been receiving support for their diagnosed eating disorder for years before their (undiagnosed) autism had been recognized.[45]

But it is clear that the underlying driving factors for autism and eating disorders are very different. In general, it matters if the autism is not spotted before an eating disorder is diagnosed, but more particularly it is likely that any treatment regimens, especially those targeting weight gain or body image problems, will miss the point. Lucy, a late-diagnosed autistic female who had spent a decade being treated for anorexia, explains:

> If you could imagine any version of hell for an autistic female, it would be being put in a grungy breakout room, stinking of the disinfectant they had swabbed the floors with after the Tumble Tots gym session. We had to sit in a circle under a flickering fluorescent light (ugh) and hold hands (double ugh) and share our eating journeys with complete strangers. Why? Just why?

Close attention to the development of disordered eating in autistic females could offer a focussed lens through which to view the consequences of their core autistic differences and how these may play out in this particular arena. So even if the answer to the question 'Is anorexia female autism?' is 'No', it is certainly worth trying to understand the reasons the question was raised in the first place.

FEMALE AUTISM AND SELF-HARM

One obvious measure of mental distress in any population is the rate of use of emergency psychiatric services. Sadly, but perhaps not unexpectedly, this appears to be greater in autistic populations, especially among girls. A survey from the Netherlands published in 2021 showed that among autistic populations referral rates to emergency psychiatric services rose from 7.9 per cent in 2009 to 18.1 per cent in 2016. The increase for adolescent girls was from 3.8 per cent to 11.1 per cent, and for boys from 14.9 per cent to 30.8 per cent.[46] Many such admissions were linked to incidences of self-harm, or NSSI.

Community-based surveys using self-report measures paint the same picture.[47] A systematic review of studies of NSSIs in autistic populations showed that, overall, they were three times more likely to self-harm than non-autistic populations.[48] A separate survey reported a prevalence estimate for self-harm in autism of 42 per cent, although it should be noted that this included self-injury arising from actions such as headbanging or eye gouging in autistic people with intellectual disabilities, as well as the cutting or scratching more commonly associated with self-harm.[49]

As with eating disorders, there are clear parallels between the profiles of those most at risk of NSSIs and those of autistic females. Taking the self-destructive aspects of NSSIs as a characteristic form of internalizing, we know that this response to psychological distress is more common in females, and especially those on the autistic spectrum. Additionally, NSSIs show a marked increase in adolescence, particularly among adolescent females.[50] Psychological risk factors include low self-esteem, high levels of anxiety, and difficulties with social interaction. An additional, telling, statistic is of higher levels of reported bullying in cases of NSSIs, so we can add frequent negative social experiences to the burden of these girls. Finally, one of the damaging consequences of camouflaging behaviour in autistic females is suicidal ideation – not NSSI per se, but as a measure of the potential for self-harm. If, then, you were asked to profile someone at high risk of self-harm, an adolescent autistic female could be the ideal candidate.

The NSSI/autism picture is slightly different from that of the overlap with eating disorders, where there are close parallels with key symptom patterns. However, the behaviour associated with the two conditions is, unless closely examined, outwardly similar. The NSSI/autism overlap appears to be linked more to the apparent choice of distress signal. Why should self-harm be more common in adolescent autistic females? The answer may lie (again) in their brains' social reward system.

Neuroscientists have proposed that the increase in NSSIs in adolescence is related to increased neural sensitivity to real or perceived social threats, which we encountered earlier in the chapter. They suggest that, paradoxically, for some individuals, self-harm, such as cutting, can reduce the impact of the response to negative social experiences.[51] According to psychological models, adolescents engage in self-harm activities to reduce or escape from the pain of social rejection, or to deal with suffering from social emotions such as shame or embarrassment. An imbalanced reward network means that the *offset* of such pain then becomes highly rewarding and the self-harming behaviour is sustained. Interviews with self-harming adolescents provide some support for this notion, with reports of reductions in depression and anxiety being associated with self-harm.[52]

So we might even be looking at a triple hit in autistic girls: self-harm is a means of alleviating the distress associated with their increasingly challenging social environment, and the relief of their social pain activates an oversensitive and maladaptive reward system. So a malfunctioning reward system comes into play here in the same way it does when driving the exaggerated responses to social rejection. Autistic females get a much greater 'hit' from self-harm than neurotypical females.

As with eating disorders, there are non-autistic individuals in the self-harming population as well as autistic. But the common factor could well be found in how individuals (and their brains) deal with negative social experiences, poor self-image, and low self-esteem. Understanding the core common mechanisms of a malfunctioning social reward system could well offer useful insights into both conditions.

FEMALE AUTISM, IDENTITY, AND GENDER DYSPHORIA

Adolescence is a time of identity change, of transition from a childhood identity determined by traditional family and social frameworks, to an independent adult identity, possibly at variance with such frameworks and expectations. This can include gender identities – the self-defined label an individual gives their gender based on their felt sense of identity. Such identities have become a matter of intense debate in recent years, with strong movements away from the traditional binary choices of being female or male (firmly fixed to biological characteristics) towards gender nonconformity and fluidity, with terms such as non-binary, gender neutral, gender fluid, and genderqueer emerging.

Many aspects of a search for a gender identity parallel those of finding an autistic identity. A consistent theme in autistic autobiographies is of being 'othered', of not belonging to your identified in-group.[53] Gender identity issues may be linked to having an identity other than that defined by your biological sex, or one that is not even within the traditional gender binary of 'female' and 'male'. There is a world full of stereotypes that are specifying what box you *should* belong in (ponder the messages that gender reveal parties might be sending out some twenty weeks or so before tiny humans even arrive on this planet). But you might feel that you don't actually fit into your assigned box, or that the residents of that particular box are telling you that you're not welcome.

Additionally, it may be that a lifetime of disguising yourself means you haven't a clear sense of your own identity, so you aren't sure where you should or want to fit anyway. Autistic females have commented that lifelong masking behaviour, constantly altering a presented persona to fit in with whatever group you're trying to identify with, has left them with a sense of having no personal identity at all. Hence, perhaps, the relief and even joy expressed when their autism diagnosis was confirmed.

Gender dysphoria, the distress caused by the incongruence between one's experienced gender and one's assigned gender, together with a persistent and strong desire to be of another gender, is a relatively rare occurrence. Estimates of the incidence can vary wildly. Some statistics, reviewed in 2009, ranged from 1:10,000 to 1:20,000 (0.01–0.005 per cent) in those assigned male at birth and 1:30,000 to 1:50,000 (0.003–0.002 per cent) in those assigned female at birth.[54] So, at that point in time, gender dysphoria was more common in those assigned male at birth. However, more recent studies (one in 2016, for example) report that the ratio has now shifted, with more adolescents assigned female at birth reporting gender dysphoria than those assigned male at birth.[55]

Although rare, interest in gender dysphoria and why and for whom it occurs is something of a hot topic at the moment, strongly linked to debates about gender identity and self-recognition. One area of note is the suggested overlap between gender dysphoria and autism. Looking at gender dysphoric populations, one study reports that 7.8 per cent of children and adolescents diagnosed with gender dysphoria were also diagnosed with ASD; another that 5.5 per cent of adults with gender dysphoria also had ASD symptoms.[56] So there is only a small percentage of individuals in each group who appear to present with both conditions (and we should remember that, with respect to gender dysphoria, we are looking at a very small population). But clinicians and researchers are hoping that exploring this area of overlap might yield some clues about identity issues in both groups.

Answers are also being sought among populations showing variations in gender identity, as opposed to clinically defined dysphoria described previously. Gender incongruence, as it is sometimes called, refers to an individual who does not feel that the gender they experience is the same as their sex assigned at birth, but who do not experience the psychological distress shown by individuals with gender dysphoria. Such variations appear to be more common in autistic populations. In 2020, a large-scale survey across five different datasets reported that transgender and gender diverse individuals were between three and six times as likely to be autistic as cisgender individuals.[57] With respect to gender identity variation in autistic populations, a survey in 2018 showed that autistic people were significantly more likely to be gender incongruent than cisgender groups.[58] And there was clear evidence that autistic individuals assigned female at birth were significantly more likely to be gender incongruent than those assigned male at birth. Autistic females were much more likely to identify outside of a gender binary, with 26.5 per cent identifying with a non-binary 'other' identity. Possibly linked to this were findings that autistic females had lower gender identification and/or lower self-esteem linked to their gender than autistic males (and also than typically developing females and males).[59] We should note that measures of nonconformity or low levels of gender identification in girls could include levels of 'tomboyism', which would include being more likely to play games associated with the opposite gender, or being more likely to imitate TV characters of the opposite sex, or being less likely to experiment with cosmetics. (You might ponder whether this tells us more about the girls or more about the expectations of the world in which they find themselves.)

A wide range of explanations has been explored for the higher levels of gender variance in autistic females, including another appearance of the extreme male brain–type link with prenatal testosterone that we saw in chapter 2 when discussing the extreme male brain theory. This suggests that females on the spectrum are more hormonally 'masculinized' and hence less strongly identified with their birth sex gender. There are some parallels with such suggestions and the findings from research into the effects of heightened levels of prenatal testosterone in girls with congenital adrenal hyperplasia (CAH).[60] As well as indications that girls with CAH are less affected by the pressures of gender socialization, as measured by toy choice or career preference for example, there are reports that this population experiences lower explicit identification with their gender group and higher incidence of gender dysphoria. However, it should also be pointed out that nearly 95 per cent of CAH girls report a female gender identity. An alternative, social explanation for gender variance in autistic females, given by Sarah Bargiela, who has offered many rich insights into the lived experiences of autistic women, is that the gender nonconformity of autistic girls could be linked to feelings of incompatibility with the traditional female role. As noted previously, this insight might tell us more about the female role than about the autistic females themselves.

Sadly, awareness of the interplay between autism and gender identity issues has some negative consequences. One worrying issue is that individuals with gender dysphoria are reporting that their concerns are somehow discredited if it also emerges that they are on the spectrum. As one autistic individual noted, 'If I happen to mention being both non-binary . . . and being autistic, people take me less seriously because they are like "oh if you are autistic, then you don't know as much"'.[61]

Another issue is that since many ASD girls have spent their lives as feeling 'other', as not being able to fit in, many are bullied for being different. Add to this mix the popular conception of autism as a male thing – even linked to an 'extreme male brain' – and girls on the spectrum may well feel that they would be 'better' aligned to a different sex – or none at all. Self-reports from autistic females often include reference to a disconnect between their gender and commonly held perceptions of autism: 'You tell someone that you're autistic and they say you're not a white, cis male. No way – you're not autistic! But you show emotion, but you're not Leonard Nimoy'.[62]

As we have seen, the drive to belong is as powerful in autistic girls as it is in typical girls, if not more so, so seeking an in-group different from the one that appears to reject them is perhaps also understandable. The hyper-femininity that currently characterizes twenty-first-century social media and marketing may also play a part. If a scan of the alleged characteristics associated with your 'assigned' identity doesn't chime with your response to what best defines you, then you may well seek a different identity altogether. If, according to gender socialization discussions, females are, on average, more powerfully driven to belong to their female in-group, then rejection by that very group would be more powerfully felt. The higher levels of gender identity nonconformity among autistic females could well be a response to this.

Another intersecting issue between gender nonconformity and autism is that of stigma. At least some expressions of gender invariance could be secondary to autism, which can lead to such expressions somehow being sidelined, or taken less seriously, as the interviewee above reported. But Jack Turban, a psychiatrist specializing in the treatment of transgender youth, has queried the strength of the link between gender dysphoria and autism, despite what the numbers appear to be saying.[63] Both conditions are associated with stigma and social rejection, which could lead to high scores on measurements of social impairment.[64] So the causality may be the other way round, with what looks like traits of autism actually being caused by the stress of social exclusion, rather than a manifestation of true autism.

Could looking at brains give any more insight into these issues? Neuroscientists are starting to compare brain connectivity profiles in individuals with both autism and gender identity diversity to explore potential areas of overlap. A 2023 study from the US looked at patterns of connectivity between the default mode network (the self-referential, daydreaming network) and other parts of the brain in forty-five transgender youth.[55] Sixteen of these were non-autistic (four identifying as female, twelve as male); fifteen were diagnosed autistic (nine identifying as female, six as male); and fourteen had high levels of autistic traits but had not been diagnosed as on the spectrum (six identified as female and eight as male). The oft-reported pattern of hyperconnectivity in the autistic group was replicated by this study. Intriguingly, levels of connectivity were higher in those designated female at birth now identifying as males. The interpretation of such findings is that there is some kind of heightened self-referencing, self-monitoring drive in the brains of transgender individuals, reflecting the ongoing quest for some kind of identity, marked both by persistent self-reflection or by repeated self-comparisons with those around you. Overall, this hyperconnectivity pattern was more closely associated with those assigned female at birth. This would be consistent with many of the other studies we have looked at, with higher levels of connectivity in parts of the social brain in autistic females, paralleling greater evidence of self- and other-monitoring in social situations. We should bear in mind that we are looking at very small numbers here. But at least the researchers were looking at gender differences!

The presence of autism in populations where gender identity is more fluid signals the need to explore issues of self-identity in autistic individuals, especially those who camouflage. Such an investigation could add a useful dimension to understanding social difficulties, arising not only from a failure to understand and follow sets of social rules, but also entangled with challenges around establishing a clear sense of self.

FEMALE AUTISM AND ADOLESCENCE: A WINDOW OF OPPORTUNITY?

It is only in the last decade or so that neuroscientists have mapped out the dramatic brain changes that occur in adolescence, and matched them with the accompanying behavioural changes. A focus on this stage of development could provide valuable insights into key aspects of how autism presents in females, as we now know that adolescence can be a very problematic phase for them. It is often during adolescence that their previously hidden problems become sufficiently evident that they may finally be identified as in need of help. But for some, their difficulties might present in ways that still allow their autism to go unnoticed, because the diagnostic dice have settled on other labels such as those we have explored here, of an eating disorder, self-harm, or gender dysphoria. Remember that group of autistic females who had all undergone years of (ineffective) treatment for eating disorders before their autism was finally revealed?

But the overlap of such conditions is at last being recognized, offering important insights into the origins and presentation of autism in women. In each of these areas – eating disorders, self-harm, and gender dysphoria – researchers continue to explore the possibility that autism brings some kind of particular susceptibility to a range of atypical behavioural patterns, perhaps because of an overlap of the genetic bases of these conditions, or perhaps because certain aspects of autism might lead to such behavioural difficulties. Are autistic women more likely to have eating disorders because of sensory problems, for example? In which case, treatment could better focus on the more fundamental sensory issues rather than assume some kind of weight phobia. It is clear that the success of treatment for eating disorders is greatly reduced when the sufferer is also autistic, so it is important that the source of the issue be correctly identified.

Might we be seeing the male spotlight at work, where clinicians focus on what they see as more common in females (eating disorders), ignoring what they think of as more common in males (autism)? What might such misdiagnoses be telling us about the reliability of the diagnostic process, particularly when we already know of its shortcomings in revealing autism in females (or not)? Gillberg's original notion, that anorexia is actually a form of female autism, has not stood the test of time. It did, however, draw attention to the possibility of co-occurring conditions, which could offer mutually useful insights into each set of differences and difficulties.[66] The fact that such co-occurrence is more common in autistic females could prove doubly beneficial to research into this hitherto under-studied group.

WHAT WE HAVE SEEN IN PART 2 OF THIS BOOK IS THAT THE MALE spotlight problem in the clinical and psychological fields of descriptions, definitions, and diagnosis of autism identified in part 1 is, if anything, even more marked in neuroscience, in research into the biological bases of autism. Until the last decade, hundreds of well-meaning investigations into the brain bases of autism have not included females at all. Newly emerging findings from studies that *do* include females are demonstrating that the 'robust' autism-related differences previously observed in autistic male-only cohorts (rarely identified as such in the research reports) do not fully generalize to autistic females. These male-biased studies have produced influential reports of patterns of underconnectivity and reduced activation in the social reward system, neatly matching the traditional, Kanner-type image of autism. But add autistic females to the equation, particularly those showing the apparently socially driven camouflaging behaviour so much at odds with the early pictures of autism, and the brain data look remarkably different. If anything, they illustrate a social brain system in overdrive, with persistent self- (and other-) monitoring accompanied by hyperconnectivity and overactivation. A radical rewrite is called for!

We should now turn our thoughts to 'where next?' We have a better view of our previously lost girls and, perhaps, have found their place on the spectrum. Now we could think about lessons learned and what the future might look like for these newly discovered members of the autism community.

CONCLUSION

ASKING BETTER QUESTIONS, GETTING BETTER ANSWERS

Autism's lost girls and women have long been overlooked, unrecognized, underdiagnosed, and left off the spectrum. In this book, we have explored what it is about this particular group of autistic people that has kept them under the autism radar for so long. I am hesitant to suggest that we may be able to sum up what we have found in a couple of phrases but basically there are two overriding explanations. Autistic girls and women went missing because no one was looking for them (the male spotlight problem) and/or because they were 'hiding' (the camouflaging problem).

The notion of camouflaging as hiding is not to imply any form of deliberate deceit, but to highlight that this pattern of behaviour, described to me so many times by autistic girls and women as a survival strategy ('I want to avoid the bullying mostly'), tells us so much about a world in which even children as young as four or five feel the need to make themselves a mask to hide behind. Moreover, they feel compelled to keep that mask in place, despite the exhaustion and stress that follow.

One of the late-diagnosed autistic women I spoke to, a health worker on the front line during the pandemic, said the relentless anxiety she felt at that time powerfully reminded her of the constant apprehension that had overshadowed her pre-diagnosis days. Another described her adult difficulties as a form of post-traumatic stress brought on by what she had suffered during her school days. We need to take a clear-eyed look at how we could make the world a better place for those who are different.

ASKING BETTER QUESTIONS: WHAT IS AUTISM?

A better question could well be, what is it like to be autistic? As we have seen, one of the breakthroughs in this story came from powerful personal testimonies from women writing about their own experiences. And these testimonies have driven an innovative change in how autism research is done, focussing on the inclusion of autistic people at all stages of the process. They can advise on the questions to ask, be involved in ensuring the recruitment will reach the right groups, and recommend adjustments to be made when devising tasks for the brain scanner, for example. In addition, they can ensure that what the researchers say about their findings is consistent with the reality of being autistic.

This innovation in autism research has been called 'participatory' research, sometimes dubbed the 'nothing about us without us' movement. It incorporates what psychologist Elizabeth Pellicano, a leader in this movement, calls 'experience-based expertise'.[1] Engaging autistic people in devising appropriate tests to quantify their everyday experiences can generate useful databases against which individual scores can be compared. It can reveal, for example, that what appears to be social avoidance is actually secondary to painful sensory experiences. Supermarkets may be 'no-go' areas not because of crowds of people but because of the bright lights and towering shelves. There is a great piece on the Thinking Person's Guide to Autism website called '30 Sensory Icks: A Checklist for Autistic and Neurodivergent People', which illustrates these sorts of issues.[2]

Kerry, a late-diagnosed autistic female who had been nonverbal until the age of six, recounted an amusing episode when she was about four years old:

> Ours was a very church-going family and the church was one of those 'everyone join in' ones. Every Sunday we all had to put on our best and go up the road. I had a tweedy coat with a prickly label in its collar that felt like someone was scratching through my neck when I put it on. Every Sunday I would scream until I had a meltdown and someone had to stay behind with me. The social worker said it was a form of social avoidance and gave my bewildered family lots of games and exercises and star charts to train me to be social. They worked at this for months and eventually beamingly reported the first successful Sunday outing. All that had happened was that I had grown out of the 'torture' coat and had inherited a beautiful soft fleece from one of my sisters. And so I went happily to church.

Adjusting diagnostic tests to better reflect what it is like to be autistic (rather than what it looks like to an observer) seems to have markedly improved the likelihood that autistic women will be spotted. Records show that the recent increases in rates of diagnosis include greater numbers of diagnosed females, including those diagnosed well into adulthood.[3] Diagnosis turns out to be particularly important for this group, who report it as an amazingly positive experience, offering some form of explanation and resolution for their lifelong difficulties. As we have heard, 'finding my tribe' is definitely a mantra in this field. It can even improve self-esteem: 'I'm a normal autistic person, not an abnormal neurotypical'.[4] One of the researchers I spoke to told me she was often taken to task by clinicians for promoting the idea that there were many troubled women whose difficulties might be associated with undiagnosed autism. It was rather huffily pointed out to her that the assessment waiting lists are long enough as it is, and that there was nothing much in the way of support mechanisms available for autistic adults anyway, at least in the UK. These clinicians showed little apparent awareness of how much importance individuals might attach to having a name for their differences.

This participatory approach is allowing researchers to harness insights from autistic lived experiences and formulate meaningful ways of gathering evidence about autistic behaviour that had not previously been captured by traditional research programmes. The search for such insights was partly what was behind one of the questions I asked the people I interviewed for this book, as I described in part 2: 'If you had a session with a brain scientist like me, what would you like me to look at?' One of the requests I received was, 'Can you show what happens in my brain when roadworks stop my school bus following its normal route?' Or, more poignantly, 'Can you show the girls in my class what happens in my brain when they call me "weirdo"?'

These insights can also inform the construction of tests that better measure the full range of autistic experiences, particularly relevant for autistic females. The most valuable of these are those that have told us about camouflaging.

Tracking the stages of camouflaging can provide a road map of key aspects of social behaviour. First of all, there is the motivation, the need to fit in. What do you have to do to make the right impression and not stand out as different? To try and blend in or generate a disguise, you need to pay close attention to social information in your world. How are the people you want to be with behaving and what changes to your own behaviour will you have to make? This 'drive to hide' is a different type of social behaviour from that captured by most traditional autism screening or diagnostic tests. As we know, it is much more common in autistic females, so focussing on it should provide a more detailed picture of their differences.

By definition, if you think about it, this aspect of the autistic experience is one of the most difficult to capture, but once you get individuals to let their guard down, they can talk you through their strategies. As a result, it is possible to generate standardized descriptions of camouflaging or masking behaviours and build up a picture of how often they are used, or in what circumstances, and/or how successful they are. As we saw in chapter 4, since about 2016 more and more tests have been devised to capture this aspect of autism, which, given that it has formed the mask that has rendered so many autistic females invisible in the past, can only be a good thing. And given the links between camouflaging and poor mental health, it is also important that ways of spotting it can be added to the autism clinicians' inventory.

And it is not just routine clinical assessments that have sprung from the study of camouflaging in autism. Sarah Bargiela, the clinical psychologist who was part of the pioneering teams who first put camouflaging on the academic map, has written a graphic novel, *Camouflage: The Hidden Lives of Autistic Women*. The book draws on her conversations with autistic women as well as her more formal research, which has been hailed as improving awareness that 'autism isn't just for men'. Such accessible texts are proving to be valuable support to newly diagnosed (or still undiagnosed) women, who see themselves and their struggles in the unfolding stories, and realize how many more masked women like them have been hiding in the shadows.

But the experiences of autism that appear to be more common in girls and women are not all about camouflaging. There is also the awareness of their struggles with different aspects of social behaviour, the very reason, perhaps, that they camouflage in the first place. A Dutch team has co-developed an Autistic Women's Experience questionnaire with autism groups recruited from specialized outpatient clinics.[5] Items that best captured the experiences of the responders included self-report items about traits such as social intuition: 'I find it difficult to imagine what it would be like to be someone else', or 'I am often the last to see the point of a joke'. And we saw how a group including psychologists Laura Hull and Will Mandy devised the GABS, a way of incorporating gender-specific enquiries into one of the key autism assessment schedules, the ADOS-2.[6] This then allowed more nuanced understanding of the nature of friendships, for example. So rather than being asked whether you had friends, or if you found it easy to make friends, you might also be asked if you had just one or two intense friends, or whether you often felt like an 'outsider'. Or whether you were particularly upset if you experienced social rejection. So we are definitely moving towards trying to generate a picture of how each autistic individual experiences the world and away from trying to match them to a preconceived (and possibly male-biased) picture of what they should look like.

If we are getting a better handle on the behavioural aspects of autism in females, what kind of progress have we made in understanding what might be going on in their brains?

ASKING BETTER QUESTIONS: SEX AND THE AUTISTIC BRAIN

From the outset of the autism story, it has been clear that autism is a brain-based disorder, but the techniques that might allow researchers to match the key patterns of atypical behaviour to 'something' in the brain were not then available. The arrival of more accessible brain-imaging techniques at the end of the 1980s should have heralded a golden age for autism brain research. Promising psychological models were in place, such as autism being linked to mindblindness, and to highly unusual ways of processing sensory information.[7] Brain imaging should have been able to put some brain 'flesh' on the behavioural 'bones': we now had the right way to ask questions about autism.

But the male spotlight problem that dogged the development of accurate and reliable measures of autism was at work in the brain-imaging field as well. The result was an era of potentially valuable but ultimately limited research into the autistic brain.[8] The male spotlight problem might have been less problematic if researchers had made clear that they were testing only males (or very few females). Yet the discussion of their findings was almost always in terms of 'autism' or 'ASD' or, for example, 'autistic youth', as though these findings would refer to the autistic population as a whole. This is what Caroline Criado Perez might refer to as the 'default male issue'.[9] Either autism was such a male problem that there was no need to consider females separately, or those females that had made it through the diagnostic barriers must, almost by definition, be so like males that, if there had been enough of them to make any comparisons, no meaningful differences would have been found. Or perhaps girls just didn't get 'real' autism?

As a reformed member of the guilty-as-charged autism research community, I would (defensively but shamefacedly) like to note that this level of nuance did not often figure in devising and running autism research studies, particularly in the early days of small-scale, single-lab studies. You were presented with the reality that there were many more male potential participants available than female, so you took what you could get and adjusted your analyses accordingly. With the advent of big datasets and multicentre research centres, these kinds of issues are starting to be overcome.

There is a strange paradox at the heart of this unmasking. As I mentioned at the very beginning of this book, I and the colleagues I worked with have often been the subject of stern reprimands from the mainstream media, as well as certain quarters of the brain research community, because of our criticisms of research into sex differences in the brain.[10] Dubbed 'sex difference deniers', we have constantly been bombarded with examples of why it is so important to study sex differences in the brain.[11] Many of these examples make reference to brain-based disorders such as Alzheimer's or Parkinson's disease, where there is evidence of the former being more common in females and the latter in males. When it comes to mental health conditions, autism is almost invariably top of the list, usually accompanied by reference to the 4:1 male:female ratio. Early rumblings in the autism research community certainly urged attention to sex differences. A paper in 2013 including many of the key players in autism research was firmly entitled, 'Biological Sex Affects the Neurobiology of Autism'.[12] So there has always been a clear message that we *must* study sex differences in the brain in order to solve the autism puzzle. And yet we weren't!

Has the recognition and inclusion of more females into autism brain research programmes given us a different (and better) picture of autistic brains? A cautious summary of contemporary research into autism (aka research including autistic women) supports what has always been considered a central aspect of the condition, that there are, indeed, difficulties with social behaviour. But it adds a very significant rider, that such difficulties manifest differently in different groups of autistic individuals. Broadly speaking, there is one group, the Kanner group, who shows the traditional pattern of social withdrawal and aloofness and an apparent lack of interest in social interaction. The majority of this group are male. Brain activity in the Kanner group is consistent with under-responsiveness in the social reward system.

The second group, the Chameleons, are characterized by highly proactive attempts to mask their autistic behaviour, possibly driven by an intense desire for social interaction and integration. The majority of this group are female. Brain activity in this group is consistent with over-responsiveness in the social reward system, linked to atypical connectivity with self-referencing, self-monitoring systems.

The discovery and measurement of camouflaging behaviour in autistic females is also proving useful to brain-imaging studies. This is particularly true where studies are targeting the social brain as a key to autistic behaviour, as the activity in this network has now been shown to vary in line with the extent of camouflaging behaviour. In high-camouflaging females engaging in social tasks, much of the activity in the social brain network is consistent with high levels of self-monitoring. You may recall, from chapter 7, the observations of the researchers looking at brain activity during self-representation tasks: 'Autistic women may engage substantial insight about their own behaviours in interpersonal and social contexts – specifically, how their behaviours impact others, gauging and managing the impressions they make on others, updating the differences between their natural and camouflaged behaviours, and how such behaviours will achieve the desired goal of being perceived as neurotypical'.[13] Sounds like the Chameleons! Autistic males, on the other hand, showed little evidence of self-monitoring activity being linked to their social reward system. So, using high or low levels of camouflaging as a grouping variable could allow brain research to develop more refined models of autism.

We must be careful not to conclude that the 'cause' of autism has been found, that we can attribute Kanner or Chameleon problems to, say, an atypical striatum or a mis-wired social reward system. Now that we know so much more about the lifelong plasticity of the human brain, we must consider that the differences in the autistic brain could be a reflection of constant negative social experiences, of being bullied and ostracized, of not fitting in. But the group differences are still intriguing.

What is it about our Chameleon group that gives them such a powerful need to belong that they will relentlessly pursue complex and exhausting (and often not very successful) camouflaging tactics, to the detriment of their own mental and physical health? Is there some kind of brain process, innate or acquired, that is driving them? Given so many of our Chameleons are female, is this brain process sex-linked in some way? These may be questions that the brain-imaging community is well-placed to consider.

BETTER QUESTIONS FOR THE FUTURE

Nowadays we can actually ask – and start to answer – really complicated questions. As well as the development of new complex number-crunching approaches made possible by greater levels of computing power, there are artificial intelligence–based machine-learning programmes that can be harnessed to interrogate enormous datasets from multicentre research initiatives (once, of course, they have topped them up with no-longer-missing female data).[14] We can add many other variables to see how they fit into the story. There could be a wide range of brain-imaging data, which could include the output from different kinds of scanning techniques, and measures of both structural characteristics, especially connectivity, and patterns of functional activity in key areas such as the reward system. There could even be measures of how good each brain is at predictive coding. Multiple behavioural measures, from a full assortment of updated autism tests (including, of course, those newly sensitive to sex and gender differences) could be added to the mix. We can add in data from genetic research and information about co-occurring physical conditions such as epilepsy or gastro-intestinal problems or sleep abnormalities, or mental health issues such as self-harm or eating disorders. Social factors such as education or socio-economic status could also be incorporated. Perhaps most useful of all, it could be possible to include the outcome of any therapeutic programmes.

If we were going to be even more ambitious in our hunt to link autistic brains with autistic behaviour we could launch large-scale longitudinal studies, prioritizing all those measures that seemed to have the strongest links to autism, perhaps focussing on key developmental stages such as adolescence, to give us an ever-richer source of information.

Machine-learning programmes could then extract detailed patterns from these many groups of different variables and potentially identify different types of combinations that fit together in meaningful ways. We could continue to ask questions about our Kanners and our Chameleons. Might differences between the volume of nerve cells, indexed by measures of grey matter, or of the connections between them, showing up as white matter, be able to distinguish between different autism subtypes? Could these differences be sex-linked in some way?

Might we soon be able to match particular patterns of brain activity with different autistic difficulties? If someone shows greater activity in the social reward system in the brain, how might we harness this information in helping them to develop useful strategies to overcome the difficulties they are having in social communication? Could we identify different areas of sensory sensitivity and pinpoint how different kinds of environments might need to be adapted to avoid sensory overload? These are all better questions that have emerged from the greater understanding of autistic behaviour and autistic brains that we now have.

IS IT TIME FOR A RETHINK? YES AND NO

There is pretty universal agreement that autism is an enormously varied condition, partly due, of course, to the ever-expanding generosity of its definition. Now that we have identified a previously unrecognized group that should be admitted to the autism community, the range of behaviours covered by the spectrum is only going to broaden. Almost since the advent of the single spectrum approach in 2013, there have been earnest discussions among clinicians and researchers, as well as autistic advocacy groups and individuals, as to whether it is time for a rethink, time to give up on a single diagnostic label for autism.[15]

As we know from chapter 5, some in the research community have expressed their frustration about the 'inadequacy of a clinical label such as "autism spectrum disorder" in the pursuit of neurobiological causes'.[16] It can be difficult to ask any meaningful research questions when the autistic people you are recruiting can present in so many different ways. Is it time to reintroduce subtypes? Simon Baron-Cohen has argued in favour of this, pointing out that it might be useful to think of the autism equivalent of type 1 and type 2 diabetes – same core problem but linked to different causes or presentations.[17] Others have argued in terms of separating out types of autistic behaviour and focussing on how to treat them, or focussing on biological characteristics, such as different genetic profiles or even different wiring patterns in the brain. I discussed this issue with a clinician, who said I should be arguing for a male-female split: 'Given you've come up with evidence of sex-related differences measured by camouflaging behaviour, why don't you propose a female autism phenotype to match what has been, to all intents and purposes, a male autism phenotype?'

The argument against the clinician's proposal has previously involved circular reasoning that if you compared diagnosed females with diagnosed males, they would be pretty much the same. The discovery of the deeply male-biased nature of the diagnostic tools themselves has obviously undermined that argument.

Then there was the argument that camouflaging was the problem. Females had been missed because they had hidden their differences and difficulties. If you 'cured' their masking, then they would hurdle over the diagnostic barriers and take their rightful place on the autism spectrum.

The focus throughout this book has obviously been on why females have been missed and the fact that once we psychologists and neuroscientists got our act together and started including females in our autism research, we saw that their autism did appear to present differently and was linked to different kinds of brain activity. So should we declare a female autism subtype, with its own tests, its own behavioural and brain-based profile?

Well – and I hope this doesn't cause you to throw this book at the wall – I think we need to be very careful about dubbing anything as 'male' or 'female'. Not least because we would be short-changing any autistic males or gender variant individuals whose autism presents in more chameleon-like fashion, in exactly the same way that females were short-changed for so long. I certainly do not want to write sex out of the autism equation altogether but given that history has shown us that focussing on a single biological characteristic of autism has limited our understanding, we should do everything we can not to make the same mistakes again.

A GENDERED WORLD MAKES A GENDERED BRAIN

In her foreword to the book *Girls and Autism: Educational, Family and Personal Perspectives,* Sophie Walker, founding leader of the Women's Equality Party, UK, writes of the struggles her autistic daughter, Grace, has in getting by in a world that does not see her, of the 'double discrimination' of being both female and autistic. She quotes Grace's own summary of what this entails:

> All girls are under immense pressure to fit in and to be a certain way according to what they are told being a girl means. It's even worse for girls with autism because they are also trying to fit in with what being a human means.[18]

I have argued elsewhere that in order to understand how brains get to be different, we need to pay attention to what is going in the world outside those brains.[19] We now know that our brains can change throughout our lives as a result of the different experiences we have, the different attitudes we encounter, the different lives we lead. There is definitely some kind of biological script behind the production of a human brain, but the social stage on which it appears has a powerful part to play in shaping its owner's successes (and failures).

My insistence that the centuries-old 'blame the brain' mantra needs to acknowledge the role of the outside world in contemporary explanations of sex and gender differences in that world has got me involved in many, many discussions about gender gaps in all sorts of organizations and the extent to which we should look at the brain-changing effects of the outside world in order to understand where these gaps come from and what we might do about them.[20] It strikes me that we could think of the apparent preponderance of males in the autistic world as a rather bizarre sort of gender gap. And that, in order to understand this gender gap, as well as looking at the brains and behaviour of autistic individuals, we should also look outside, at the world that seems to impact the owners of such brains so differently and from which they so often feel excluded.

One of my ongoing campaigns is to draw attention to the role of gender in the study of the brain beyond autism. There has been quite a push in recent years to ensure that sex differences are measured in all aspects of neuroscience – the Sex as a Biological Variable movement (although this directive seems to have passed by certain fields of neuroscience!).[21] But brain-changing gendered attitudes and expectations are among the most powerful sets of experiences any of us will encounter, so I am pushing for a Gender as a Biological Variable movement. This could include both grouping variables linked to gender identity – particularly relevant to the autism community with its high levels of gender variance – but also grouping gendered 'life variables', such as, sadly, experience of intimate partner violence or abusive relationships, again considerably more prevalent among both women and the autism community, and, of course, autistic women.[22]

Looking at social context could be especially telling in autism research. One of the outside influences on the brain that social cognitive neuroscience has explored is that of negative social experiences such as bullying or rejection, a constant theme in many of the discussions I've had with autistic people. And the very brain mechanisms that swing into action in the face of such nastiness are the mechanisms that best seem to distinguish our Chameleons from our Kanners. We brain imagers could do so much better by our autistic sisters by answering the questions they want asked.

This complex question about the interaction between autism and our world brings us back to camouflaging. We know that the majority of autistic camouflagers are female. We also know that the process of camouflaging appears to have a very detrimental effect on many, if not most, of these camouflagers. And yet they persist. The reason for this is often described as some kind of survival mechanism, a wish to avoid being stigmatized and othered. It is not only autistic females who experience such unpleasantness in their world, but it is, on the whole, more likely to be autistic females who are driven into hiding. So, as well as exploring the 'how' and the 'who' of camouflaging, we should look to the role of gender in explaining the 'why'. And that should include why it is more common in females – is camouflaging linked to some sex-based mechanism that prioritizes 'belongingness'? Or could such a mechanism be acquired, given the pressures and socialization that women and girls face?[23] Back to the brain-imaging community to find ways of asking such questions – perhaps to make up for those missing female datasets in the early years of autism research!

In discussions of autism's gender gap, there have often been references to gendered differences in socialization, speculating that a greater emphasis on social niceties – on compliance and conformity – produced the 'quieter' form of autism allegedly more characteristic of autistic females. So much quieter, indeed, that it often fails to register as autism at all. We now know that the passive, shy façade might well be disguising potent levels of distress. And being on the lookout for this particular 'good girls don't' stereotype in our gendered world might mean that all those autistic girls and women, all those 'Alices', all those Chameleons, are spotted earlier. More and more, society is waking up to how gender stereotyping can negatively impact us all, particularly in the early years. Energetic initiatives are urging all those involved, from teachers to marketing gurus to policymakers, to tackle the issues around the limitations imposed by gendered expectations.[24] We should add the story of female autism to this list, to give powerful examples of how a world's expectations can drive vulnerable groups underground, to suffer unnoticed.

SOLVING THE DOUBLE EMPATHY PROBLEM

Damian Milton, an autistic academic and researcher, has identified a 'double empathy' problem in autism, a mutual lack of understanding between autistic and non-autistic individuals.[25] Autistic people can find it hard to figure out what non-autistic people are thinking and feeling, and how to work out the invisible rules that tell you how to fit in, how to be accepted, how to belong to social groups. But it is clear that non-autistic people have the same problem.[26] A combination of impressions from misleading stereotypes and few opportunities to engage fully with autistic individuals means that non-autistic people don't know what it is like to experience the world differently, to have overwhelming and genuinely painful responses to sensations that most of us can ignore or don't even notice. They will be blissfully unaware that friendly, relaxed, spontaneous social exchanges, effortlessly governed by automatically acquired invisible rules, can be experienced by autistic people as the equivalent of being parachuted into a foreign country as an undercover agent, with no understanding of the language or the local customs. They might not understand the dread caused when plans are changed at the last minute, when a whole new tranche of panic-inducing 'what if' scenarios will be triggered. They might not understand that autistic people may not have the equivalent of a 'whatever' mental shrug.

If we are going to work towards solving this two-way communication problem, then all of us – teachers, researchers, clinicians, autism advocates, and the wider public – need to get the full picture of what it is to be autistic. Neurotypical people such as myself need to hear about the lived experiences of people such as Alice, from their side of the looking glass, so we can see their world through their eyes rather than only ours. We must find the flaws that have allowed us to lose sight of these lost girls, we must challenge the fuzzy and imprecise diagnoses, and we must confront the gender stereotypes that are distorting our quest for answers in the world of autism. Maybe we can (gently) deconstruct the elaborate camouflages that have allowed autistic girls to 'fly beneath the radar', to 'hide in plain sight'.[27] We must listen to these lost girls so that autism researchers, autism therapists, autism advocates, and the wider general population will have a much clearer idea of what we should be looking for, what we need to explain, so that we can better understand the autistic world.[28]

From the other side of the looking glass, by understanding female autism, we could learn about ourselves, about the human race's overpowering desire to belong. We can unpick the intricacies of the social scripts that fulfil this need – invisible to us, but painstakingly detected by our autistic sisters. We could listen to what they have to say and realize how many different ways there are of experiencing our world. We could also understand the need to be other-aware as well as self-aware, and realize the hugely negative impact of stigmatizing and ostracizing individuals who don't fit into our one-size-fits-all expectations.

We have explored the many reasons why girls and women have been missing in the history of autism, and why it matters. We have found our way behind their masks and spotted their differently different autistic behaviour. We have finally welcomed them into our scanners and mapped their differently different brains. Hopefully we can now make the world a better place for them.

OTHER STORIES FROM BEHIND THE MASK

THE AIM OF THIS BOOK WAS TO DISCOVER THE SCIENCE behind the stories of autistic women. This pursuit introduced me to a treasure trove of personal testimonies from women who had somehow negotiated the journey towards an autism diagnosis. A mix of frustration and inspiration, often sad, frequently funny, they provided so many of the questions I hoped to answer. You will find snippets of these testimonies incorporated into *The Lost Girls of Autism*, so I'm acknowledging these women's contributions by sharing this list.

If you want to find out what it is really like to be one of autism's lost girls, to be a woman who is (or should be) on the spectrum, then any or all of these books are essential reading. My apologies if I have left off any of your favourites – please let me know so I can keep adding to this wonderful list.

Baird, Francesca. *Label Me: My Journey towards an Autism Diagnosis*. Indigo State. 2021.

Bargiela, Sarah. *Camouflage: The Hidden Lives of Autistic Women*. Jessica Kingsley Publishers. 2019.

Belcher, Hannah Louise. *Taking Off the Mask: Practical Exercises to Help Understand and Minimise the Effects of Autistic Camouflaging*. Jessica Kingsley. 2022.

Brady, Fern. *Strong Female Character*. Brazen. 2023.

Cook, Barb, and Michelle Garnett, eds. *Spectrum Women: Walking to the Beat of Autism*. Jessica Kingsley. 2018. (Not strictly an autobiographical text, this edited set of chapters is rich with many lived experience insights from autistic women.)

Davide-Rivera, Jeannie. *Twirling Naked in the Streets and No One Noticed: Growing Up with Undiagnosed Autism*. David and Goliath. 2012.

Del Vecchio, Marie-Laure, and Joe James. *The Autistic Experience: Silenced Voices Finally Heard*. Sheldon. 2023.

Gibbs, Sara. *Drama Queen: One Autistic Woman and a Life of Unhelpful Labels*. Headline. 2021.

Hendrickx, Sarah. *Women and Girls with Autism Spectrum Disorder: Understanding Life Experiences from Early Childhood to Old Age*. Jessica Kingsley. 2015. (Again, although not strictly an autobiographical testimony, this is a treasure trove of many personal experiences of autistic women and of the families of autistic girls.)

James, Laura. *Odd Girl Out: An Autistic Woman in a Neurotypical World*. Seal. 2017.

Katy, Emily. *Girl Unmasked: How Uncovering My Autism Saved My Life*. Monoray. 2024.

Kim, Cynthia. *Nerdy, Shy, and Socially Inappropriate: A User Guide to an Asperger Life*. Jessica Kingsley. 2014.

Kurchak, Sarah. *I Overcame My Autism and All I Got Was This Lousy Anxiety Disorder: A Memoir*. Douglas & McIntyre. 2020.

Lamanna, Jodi. *Arriving Late: The Lived Experience of Women Receiving a Late Autism Diagnosis*. Jessica Kingsley. 2024.

Limburg, Joanne. *Letters to My Weird Sisters: On Autism and Feminism*. Atlantic. 2021.

Nerenberg, Jenara. *Divergent Mind: Thriving in a World that Wasn't Designed for You*. HarperOne. 2020.

O'Toole, Jennifer Cook. *Autism in Heels: The Untold Story of a Female Life on the Spectrum*. Skyhorse. 2018.

Pang, Camilla. *Explaining Humans: What Science Can Teach Us about Life, Love and Relationships*. Viking. 2020.

Poe, Charlotte Amelia. *How to Be Autistic*. Myriad. 2019.

Price, Devon. *Unmasking Autism: The Power of Embracing Our Hidden Neurodiversity*. Hachette UK. 2022. (Devon Price is a trans man and does not currently identify as a woman.)

Törnvall, Clara. *The Autists: Women on the Spectrum*. Scribe. 2023.

Wells, Katy. *The Painted Clown: One Teenage Girl's Experience of Autism and Masking*. Katy Wells. 2022.

Willey, Liane Holliday. *Pretending to Be Normal: Living with Asperger's Syndrome (Autism Spectrum Disorder)*, Expanded Edition. Jessica Kingsley. 2014.

Williams, Donna. *Nobody Nowhere: The Remarkable Autobiography of an Autistic Girl*. Jessica Kingsley. 2009.

ACKNOWLEDGEMENTS

I WOULD LIKE TO THANK ALL OF THOSE WHO GAVE SO GENEROUSLY and patiently of their time in helping me find my way to and through this book (and, hopefully, out of the other side).

Firstly, thank you to those who shared their experiences of what it is like to be autistic or, more accurately, to be themselves. You shared many thought-provoking examples of how difficult life in the looking-glass world of autism can be for you, but also rather awe-inspiring insights into the invisible social rules that govern everyday life for us humans. You were also helpful in (very) politely pointing out some of my own 'blind spots' in my understanding of autism – and helpfully suggesting reading material (especially thank you to those who introduced me to Elle McNicoll's great books – I've read them all now!). The emerging involvement of you and your autistic colleagues in future autism research activities will continue to transform the questions we researchers should be asking – and, hopefully, the answers we will be getting.

Secondly, there were parents, siblings, carers, teachers, support workers, advocates, and friends who shared their insights into the autistic experience from the other side of the looking glass, as it were, but who clearly had their noses pressed closest to it. Your patience, generosity, and understanding as well as, quite often, your pride in those negotiating a world that all too often fails to understand them, has been quite overwhelming at times.

While all of you were generous (and brave) enough to share your stories with me and for these to inform the pages of this book, some of you did not wish to be named or be identifiable. Therefore, names have been altered and stories have been edited to ensure as much anonymity as possible. With this in mind, I will not list my interviewees here – you know who you are and how grateful I am. I hope I have accurately represented your thoughts and concerns in this book and that you genuinely feel part of what I hope will be a step forward to a better future for you all. THANK YOU!

That having been said, there are three special people who comprised a particular dream team for my quest, who can be named. They are already well known as scientists and science writers, and each of them has publicly shared their experiences of being on the autism spectrum (you see what I mean by dream team). So, to Hannah Belcher, Sue Nelson, and Camilla Pang, thank you for your time and valuable conversations.

In addition to these many opportunities to gain some personal insights into the world of autistic experiences (as opposed, I have to confess, to just mulling over the outputs from brain-imaging studies), I benefited greatly from the many powerful testimonies written by courageous autistic women, very few of whom had been recognized as autistic in their early years, with most not diagnosed until well into their twenties, thirties, or even beyond. I have listed some of their books after the final chapter. Thank you all for finding your voices and using them so effectively.

There are several key researchers who are already striving to counteract the male bias in the autism research arena, many of whom generously gave up their time to speak with me or take a Zoom call, to talk me through their work in this field and make helpful suggestions about what the book should try to cover. Some of them seem to figure on just about every paper on female autism there is, so it was a privilege to talk to them. Thank you, then, and much respect to Francesca Happé, Laura Hull, Meng-Chuan Lai, Will Mandy, Ralph-Axel Müller, Liz Pellicano, and Felicity Sedgewick. Sarah-Jayne Blakemore offered helpful advice on adolescence, and I had a very fruitful email exchange of views with Simon Baron-Cohen about the current state of autism diagnosis and assessment.

My own autism research journey began with the support of Jill Boucher, Jon Brock, and Caroline Brown, for which many thanks. Jon was also the creator of the Zap the Aliens task, and he and the MEG imaging staff at Macquarie University in Sydney were immensely supportive of the road testing of the task while I was on sabbatical there. Back at Aston, the work continued with Klaus Kessler and Robert Seymour, with whom I enjoyed many stimulating 'predictive coding' discussions, as well as too many cups of Klaus's even more stimulating espressos. The MEG team here, as ever, were amazing.

Behind the scenes in getting this book to the finishing line, I must offer special thanks to Kate Barker, my agent, who encouraged me to write a book about women and autism in the first place, and who has been a tireless advisor, path-smoother, and rant-absorber throughout. Having found myself in the outside world of science writing (again, thanks to Kate) and shared 'agents' tales' with other authors, I realize how lucky I am. Helen Edwards also worked hard to find the US partners for me – thank you very much.

I must thank my editors, of whom, for various reasons, there have been several! Janice Audet from Seal Press in the US was extremely understanding and helpful with the first draft and carried on refining and improving several of the next rounds, right up until midnight, I do believe, on the day before she left for pastures new. She was richly aided and abetted by Madeline Lee, who also moved on, but left me a rich legacy of helpful insights. Emily Taber then 'inherited' me and has proved a calm sounding board in the closing stages. Mike Harpley, of Pan Macmillan, has steered and steadied the ship from the other side of the Atlantic; this book would have been a very different beast without him. Copy editor Lillian Duggan had the unenviable job of scrutinizing my final text; apologies for the hard work I caused you, Lillian, and thank you for your patient and polite queries and corrections. The production team on both sides of the Atlantic are already going great guns so thank you in advance. Thank you all for your time and input – I could not do what you do (which may well have been obvious throughout!).

There has been an amazing series of backup teams throughout my academic and writing career, who have been both clear-eyed critical friends and supportive sympathizers. First and foremost these include my good friends and colleagues the non-Davids (Lise Eliot, Cordelia Fine, Daphna Joel, and Donna Maney), who are leaders in sex/gender debates beyond autism, and whose fierce fileting of inadequate thinking has saved me from many an elephant trap. We owe each other another Santa Fe retreat!

In the same vein, fellow members of the NeuroGenderings board have had each other's backs through recent tough times, but I believe we have managed never to lose sight of our core mission, to develop better approaches for gender-informed research. This includes helpful updates for people like me struggling to find our way through cross-disciplinary minefields. I would particularly like to mention Robyn Bluhm, Katherine Bryant, Annie Duchesne, Hannah Fitsch, Giordana Grossi, Beck Jordan-Young, Anelis Kaiser, and Sigrid Schmitz. Please keep up the good work.

I sadly only found out about the Neuwrite London network after writing *The Gendered Brain*. This network of science writers and journalists workshop each other's pieces for publication but also cheer on each other when the going gets tough. We also go to each other's book launches, which, when you've turned into a writing hermit, may be the only time we see daylight outside our studies/cubby-holes/kitchen tables. Publicists, please note. Thank you, then, to my fellow Neuwriters, Roma Agrawal, Yasmin Ali, Hana Ayoob, Subhadra Das, Rageshri Dhairywan, Anjana Khatwa, Alex O'Brien, Paula Rowińska, and others, all of whom have written amazing science books but have made time to comment on mine.

Angela Saini has also been linked to Neuwrite as well as being active in the very helpful Association of British Science Writers and, more particularly, in founding the Challenging Pseudoscience network. Her books *Inferior, Superior*, and, most recently, *The Patriarchs*, have been an envy-inducing source of fascinating insights into the consequences of the kind of gendered lens that has distorted the autism story to date. Additionally, her personal support for my various writing and researching activities has been invaluable. She also let me 'borrow' one of her subtitles, and treated me to cocktails in New York, so extra thanks are due.

As with *The Gendered Brain*, there would not have been any book at all for which to thank these wonderful people had it not been for Dennis. He has seen me through the many downs, and the rather fewer ups, on the road to this point. He has been patient as ever, stoically altering travel plans and postponing holidays. He must dread those four words: 'This won't take long'. To Dennis, then, along with daughters Anna and Eleanor, I'm sorry I've been 'away' but I am back again now. Thank you for looking after me.

NOTES

PREFACE. WHY ME AND WHY THIS BOOK?

1. Cleghorn, E. (2022). *Unwell women: Misdiagnosis and myth in a man-made world*. Penguin; Criado Perez, C. (2019). *Invisible women: Data bias in a world designed for men*. Vintage; Rippon, G. (2019). *The gendered brain: The new neuroscience that shatters the myth of the female brain*. Random House.

2. World Health Organization. *Sexual health*. www.who.int/health-topics/sexual-health#tab=tab_2.

3. World Health Organization Europe. *Gender*. www.who.int/europe/health-topics/gender#tab=tab_1.

4. World Health Organization. *Gender and health*. www.who.int/health-topics/gender#tab=tab_1.

5. World Health Organization. *Gender and health*. www.who.int/health-topics/gender#tab=tab_1.

6. Walsh, R. J., Krabbendam, L., Dewinter, J., & Begeer, S. (2018). Brief report: Gender identity differences in autistic adults: Associations with perceptual and socio-cognitive profiles. *Journal of autism and developmental disorders, 48*(12), 4070–8.

7. Lord, C., Charman, T., Havdahl, A., Carbone, P., Anagnostou, E., Boyd, B., Carr, T., de Vries, P. J., Dissanayake, C., Divan, G., et al. (2022). The Lancet Commission on the future of care and clinical research in autism. *Lancet, 399*, 271–334.

8. Kapp, S. K. (2023). Profound concerns about 'profound autism': Dangers of severity scales and functioning labels for support needs. *Education Sciences, 13*(2), 106; but also see Singer, S. (2022, October 27). *It's time to embrace 'profound autism'*. The Transmitter. www.thetransmitter.org/spectrum/its-time-to-embrace-profound-autism.

INTRODUCTION

1. World Health Organization. (2023, November). *Autism* [Fact sheet]. www.who.int/news-room/fact-sheets/detail/autism-spectrum-disorders.

2. Maenner, M. J., Warren, Z., Williams, A. R., et al. (2023). Prevalence and characteristics of autism spectrum disorder among children aged 8 years – Autism and developmental disabilities monitoring network, 11 sites, United

States, 2020. *MMWR Surveillance Summaries*, 72(SS-2), 1–14. www.cdc.gov/mmwr/volumes/72/ss/ss7202a1.htm?s_cid=ss7202a1_w.

3. Roman-Urrestarazu, A., Yang, J. C., van Kessel, R., Warrier, V., Dumas, G., Jongsma, H., Gatica-Bahamonde, G., Allison, C., Matthews, F. E., Baron-Cohen, S., & Brayne, C. (2022). Autism incidence and spatial analysis in more than 7 million pupils in English schools: A retrospective, longitudinal, school registry study. *The Lancet Child & Adolescent Health*, 6(12), 857–68.

4. Whitlock, A., Fulton, K., Lai, M.-C., Pellicano, E., & Mandy, W. (2020). Recognition of girls on the autism spectrum by primary school educators: An experimental study. *Autism Research*, *13*(8), 1358–72.

5. Kanner, L. (1943). Autistic disturbances of affective contact. *Nervous Child*, *2*, 217–50.

6. Wing, L. (1981). Sex ratios in early childhood autism and related conditions. *Psychiatry Research*, 5(2), 129–37.

CHAPTER 1. WHAT IS AUTISM?

1. Happé, F., & Frith, U. (2020). Annual Research Review: Looking back to look forward – changes in the concept of autism and implications for future research. *Journal of Child Psychology and Psychiatry*, *61*(3), 218–32; Mandy, W. (2023). The old and the new way of understanding autistic lives: Reflections on the life of Donald Triplett, the first person diagnosed as autistic. *Autism*, *27*(7), 1853–5; Donald Triplett obituary. (2023, July 31). *The Times*. www.thetimes.com/uk/obituaries/article/donald-triplett-obituary-dnx72bk6r; Kent Presents. (2018, November 9). *In a Different Key: The Story of Autism* [Video]. YouTube. www.youtube.com/watch?v=CjwwFIJdUXc.

2. Carroll, L. (1872). *Through the looking-glass, and what Alice found there*. Macmillan.

3. Bleuler, E. (1911). *Dementia praecox or the group of schizophrenias*. International Universities Press.

4. 'Refrigerator mothers' was a psychoanalytical theory of autism espoused by Bruno Bettelheim, that autism was caused by a lack of maternal affection; by cold, distant, and rejecting mothers. Popular in the 1950s and 1960s, it fell out of favour once more biological explanations emerged.

5. Kanner, L. (1943). Autistic disturbances of affective contact. *Nervous Child*, *2*, 217–50.

6. Asperger, H. (1944). Die 'autistischen psychopathen' im kindesalter. *Archiv für Psychiatrie und Nervenkrakheiten*, *117*, 76–136.

7. American Psychiatric Association and National Committee for Mental Hygiene (1918). *Statistical Manual for the Use of Institutions for the Insane*. National Committee for Mental Hygiene, Bureau of Statistics.

8. Surís, A., Holliday, R., & North, C. S. (2016). The evolution of the classification of psychiatric disorders. *Behavioral Sciences*, 6(1), 5; Gurland,

B. J., Fleiss, J. L., Cooper, J. E., Sharpe, L., Kendell, R. E., & Roberts, P. (1970). Cross-national study of diagnosis of mental disorders: Hospital diagnoses and hospital patients in New York and London. *Comprehensive Psychiatry, 11*, 18–25.

9. American Psychiatric Association. (2013). *Diagnostic and statistical manual of mental disorders, fifth edition: DSM-5*. American Psychiatric Association.

10. Rimland, B. (1968). On the objective diagnosis of infantile autism. *Acta Paedopsychiatrica, 35*, 146–61; Parks, S. L. (1983). The assessment of autistic children: A selective review of available instruments. *Journal of Autism and Developmental Disorders, 13*(3), 255–67.

11. Creak, M. (1961). Schizophrenic syndrome in childhood: Progress report of a working party. *Cerebral Palsy Bulletin, 3*, 501–4.

12. American Psychiatric Association. (1980). *Diagnostic and statistical manual of mental disorders, third edition: DSM-3*. American Psychiatric Association.

13. Wing, L. & Gould, J. (1979). Severe impairments of social interaction and associated abnormalities in children: Epidemiology and classification. *Journal of Autism and Developmental Disorders, 9*(1), 11–29.

14. Wing, L. (1981). Asperger's syndrome: A clinical account. *Psychological Medicine, 11*(1), 115–29.

15. Wing, L. (2005). Reflections on opening Pandora's box. *Journal of Autism and Developmental Disorders, 35*(2), 197–203.

16. Asperger, H. (1991). 'Autistic psychopathy' in childhood. In U. Frith (Ed.), *Autism and Asperger syndrome* (pp. 37–92). Cambridge University Press.

17. American Psychiatric Association. (1994). *Diagnostic and statistical manual of mental disorders, fourth edition: DSM-4*. American Psychiatric Association.

18. Thunberg, G. [@GretaThunberg]. (2019, August 31). *When haters go after your looks and differences . . .* [Post]. X. https://x.com/GretaThunberg/status/1167916177927991296?lang=en.

19. Lime Connect. (2016, March 23). *Interview with Dr. Stephen Shore: Autism advocate & on the spectrum*. International Board of Credentialing and Continuing Education Standards. https://ibcces.org/blog/2018/03/23/12748.

20. Volkmar, F. R., & McPartland, J. C. (2014). From Kanner to DSM-5: Autism as an evolving diagnostic concept. *Annual Review of Clinical Psychology, 10*(1), 93–212.

21. Grinker, R. R. (2007). *Unstrange minds: Remapping the world of autism*. Basic Books.

22. Leekam, S. R., Prior, M. R., & Uljarevic, M. (2011). Restricted and repetitive behaviors in autism spectrum disorders: A review of research in the last decade. *Psychological Bulletin, 137*(4), 562.

23. Wrong Planet. https://wrongplanet.net.

24. World Health Organization. (2022). International statistical classification of diseases and related health problems (10th ed.). https://icd.who.int/en.

25. Hartwell, M., Keener, A., Coffey, S., Chesher, T., Torgerson, T., & Vassar, M. (2021). Brief report: Public awareness of Asperger syndrome following Greta Thunberg appearances. *Journal of Autism and Developmental Disorders, 51*(6), 2104–8.

26. Kanner, L. (1943). Autistic disturbances of affective contact. *Nervous Child, 2*, 217–50.

27. Lord, C., Rutter, M., DiLavore, P., et al. (2002). Autism diagnostic observation scale. Western Psychological Services; Rutter, M., Le Couteur, A., & Lord, C. (2003). Autism diagnostic interview – revised. Western Psychological Services.

28. Constantino, J. N., Davis, S. A., Todd, R. D., Schindler, M. K., Gross, M. M., Brophy, S. L., Metzger, L. M., Shoushtari, C. S., Splinter, R., & Reich, W. (2003). Validation of a brief quantitative measure of autistic traits: Comparison of the social responsiveness scale with the autism diagnostic interview – revised. *Journal of Autism and Developmental Disorders, 33*, 427–33.

CHAPTER 2. AUTISM'S MALE SPOTLIGHT PROBLEM

1. Barsky, R. F. (1998). *Noam Chomsky: A life of dissent* (reprint ed.). MIT Press.

2. Asperger, H. (1991). 'Autistic psychopathy' in childhood. In U. Frith (Ed.), *Autism and Asperger syndrome* (pp. 37–92). Cambridge University Press.

3. Sheffer, E. (2018). *Asperger's children: The origins of autism in Nazi Vienna*. W. W. Norton & Company.

4. Sheffer, E. (2018). *Asperger's children: The origins of autism in Nazi Vienna*. W. W. Norton & Company; Asperger, H. (1991). 'Autistic psychopathy' in childhood. In U. Frith (Ed.), *Autism and Asperger syndrome* (pp. 37–92). Cambridge University Press.

5. Sheffer, E. (2018). *Asperger's children: The origins of autism in Nazi Vienna*. W. W. Norton & Company.

6. Czech, H. (2018). Hans Asperger, National Socialism, and 'race hygiene' in Nazi-era Vienna. *Molecular Autism, 9*, 29; Sher, D. A. (2020, July 27). *The aftermath of the Hans Asperger exposé*. The British Psychological Society. www.bps.org.uk/psychologist/aftermath-hans-asperger-expose.

7. Sheffer, E. (2018). *Asperger's children: The origins of autism in Nazi Vienna*. W. W. Norton & Company.

8. Sheffer, E. (2018). *Asperger's children: The origins of autism in Nazi Vienna*. W. W. Norton & Company.

9. Asperger, H. (1991). 'Autistic psychopathy' in childhood. In U. Frith (Ed.), *Autism and Asperger syndrome* (pp. 37–92). Cambridge University Press.

10. Baron-Cohen, S., Klin, A., Silberman, S., & Buxbaum, J. D. (2018). Did Hans Asperger actively assist the Nazi euthanasia program? *Molecular Autism, 9*, 1–2.

11. Ssucharewa, G. E. (1926). Die schizoiden Psychopathien im Kindesalter. *Monatsschrift für Psychiatrie und Neurologie, 60*, 235–61; Rebecchi, K. (2022). *Autistic children: Grunya Efimovna Sukhareva*. Kevin Rebecchi.

12. Wolff, S. (1996). The first account of the syndrome Asperger described? Translation of a paper entitled 'Die schizoiden Psychopathien im Kindesalter' by Dr G. E. Ssucharewa. *European Society of Child and Adolescent Psychiatry, 5*, 119–32.

13. Manouilenko, I., & Bejerot, S. (2015). Sukhareva – Prior to Asperger and Kanner. *Nordic Journal of Psychiatry, 69*, 1761–4.

14. Posar, A., & Visconti, P. (2017). Tribute to Grunya Efimovna Sukhareva, the woman who first described infantile autism. *Journal of Pediatric Neuroscience, 12*, 300–1.

15. Simmonds, C., & Sukhareva, G. E. (2020). The first account of the syndrome Asperger described? Part 2: The girls. *European Child & Adolescent Psychiatry, 29*(4), 549–64.

16. Rebecchi, K. (2022). *Autistic children: Grunya Efimovna Sukhareva*. Kevin Rebecchi.

17. Sher, D. A., & Gibson, J. L. (2023). Pioneering, prodigious and perspicacious: Grunya Efimovna Sukhareva's life and contribution to conceptualising autism and schizophrenia. *European Child & Adolescent Psychiatry, 32*, 475–90. https://doi.org/10.1007/s00787-021-01875-7.

18. Szalavitz, M. (2016, February). The invisible girls. *Scientific American Mind, 27*(2), 48–55. www.jstor.org/stable/24945379.

19. Kanner, L. (1955). Infantile autism. In S. Arieti (Ed.), *American Handbook of Psychiatry: Volume One* (pp. 556–81). Basic Books.

20. Lotter, V. (1966). Epidemiology of autistic conditions in young children. I. Prevalence. *Social Psychiatry, 1*, 124–37.

21. Wing, L., & Gould, J. (1979). Severe impairments of social interaction and associated abnormalities in children: Epidemiology and classification. *Journal of Autism and Developmental Disorders, 9*(1), 1–29.

22. Wing, L. (1981). Sex ratios in early childhood autism and related conditions. *Psychiatry Research, 5*(2), 129–37.

23. Ehlers, S., & Gillberg, C. (1993). The epidemiology of Asperger syndrome: A total population study. *Journal of Child Psychology and Psychiatry, 34*(8), 1327–50.

24. Posserud, M.-B., Skretting Solberg, B., Engeland, A., Haavik, J., & Klungsøyr, K. (2021). Male to female ratios in autism spectrum disorders by age, intellectual disability and attention-deficit/hyperactivity disorder. *Acta Psychiatrica Scandinavica, 144*(6), 635–46.

25. Loomes, R., Hull, L., & Mandy, W. P. L. (2017). What is the male-to-female ratio in autism spectrum disorder? A systematic review and meta-analysis. *Journal of the American Academy of Child and Adolescent Psychiatry, 56*(6), 466–74.

26. Zeidan, J., Fombonne, E., Scorah, J., Ibrahim, A., Durkin, M. S., Saxena, S., Yusuf, A., Shih, A., & Elsabbagh, M. (2022). Global prevalence of autism: A systematic review update. *Autism Research, 15*(5), 778–90.

27. Lockwood Estrin, G., Milner, V., Spain, D., Happé, F., & Colvert, E. (2021). Barriers to autism spectrum disorder diagnosis for young women and girls: A systematic review. *Review Journal of Autism and Developmental Disorders, 8*(4), 454–70.

28. Russell, G., Golding, J., Norwich, B., Emond, A., Ford, T., & Steer, C. (2012). Social and behavioural outcomes in children diagnosed with autism spectrum disorders: A longitudinal cohort study. *Journal of Child Psychology and Psychiatry, 53*(7), 735–44.

29. Szalavitz, M. (2016, February). The invisible girls. *Scientific American Mind, 27*(2), 48–55. www.jstor.org/stable/24945379.

30. Russell, G., Steer, C., & Golding, J. (2011). Social and demographic factors that influence the diagnosis of autistic spectrum disorders. *Social Psychiatry and Psychiatric Epidemiology, 46*(12), 1283–93.

31. Whitlock, A., Fulton, K., Lai, M.-C., Pellicano, E., & Mandy, W. (2020). Recognition of girls on the autism spectrum by primary school educators: An experimental study. *Autism Research, 13*(8), 1358–72.

32. Duvekot, J., van der Ende, J., Verhulst, F. C., Slappendel, G., van Daalen, E., Maras, A., & Greaves-Lord, K. (2017). Factors influencing the probability of a diagnosis of autism spectrum disorder in girls versus boys. *Autism, 21*(6), 646–58.

33. Kaat, A. J., Shui, A. M., Ghods, S. S., Farmer, C. A., Esler, A. N., Thurm, A., Georgiades, S., Kanne, S. M., Lord, C., Kim, Y. S., & Bishop, S. L. (2021). Sex differences in scores on standardized measures of autism symptoms: A multisite integrative data analysis. *Journal of Child Psychology and Psychiatry, 62*(1), 97–106.

34. Ratto, A. B. (2021). Commentary: What's so special about girls on the autism spectrum? – A commentary on Kaat et al. (2020). *Journal of Child Psychology and Psychiatry, 62*(1), 107–9.

35. McCrossin R. (2022). Finding the true number of females with autistic spectrum disorder by estimating the biases in initial recognition and clinical diagnosis. *Children (Basel), 9*(2), 272.

36. D'Mello, A. M., Frosch, I. R., Li, C. E., Cardinaux, A. L., & Gabrieli, J. D. (2022). Exclusion of females in autism research: Empirical evidence for a 'leaky' recruitment-to-research pipeline. *Autism Research, 15*(10), 1929–40.

37. Di Martino, A., Yan, C.-G., Li, Q., Denio, E., Castellanos, F. X., Alaerts,

K., Anderson, J. S., Assaf, M., Bookheimer, S. Y., Dapretto, M., Deen, B., et al. (2014). The autism brain imaging data exchange: Towards a large-scale evaluation of the intrinsic brain architecture in autism. *Molecular Psychiatry, 19*(6), 659–67.

38. Baron-Cohen, S. (2002). The extreme male brain theory of autism. *Trends in Cognitive Sciences, 6*(6), 248–54.

39. Eliot, L., Ahmed, A., Khan, H., & Patel, J. (2021). Dump the 'dimorphism': Comprehensive synthesis of human brain studies reveals few male-female differences beyond size. *Neuroscience & Biobehavioral Reviews, 125*, 667–97.

40. Joel, D., Berman, Z., Tavor, I., Wexler, N., Gaber, O., Stein, Y., Shefi, N., Pool, J., Urchs, S., Margulies, D. S., Liem, F., et al. (2015). Sex beyond the genitalia: The human brain mosaic. *Proceedings of the National Academy of Sciences, 112*(50), 15468–73.

41. Rippon, G. (2019). *The gendered brain: The new neuroscience that shatters the myth of the female brain*. Random House.

42. Ridley, R. (2019). Some difficulties behind the concept of the 'extreme male brain' in autism research. A theoretical review. *Research in Autism Spectrum Disorders, 57*, 19–27.

43. Baron-Cohen, S. (2004). *The essential difference: Male and female brains and the truth about autism*. Penguin UK.

44. Baron-Cohen, S. (2020). *The pattern seekers: A new theory of human invention*. Penguin UK.

45. Offord, J. (Host). (2020, November 24). A conversation with Simon Baron-Cohen [Audio podcast episode]. In *The Different Minds*. https://creators.spotify.com/pod/show/differentminds/episodes/A-conversation-with-Simon-Baron-Cohen-emudeb/a-a3ujdj6.

46. Gillis-Buck, E., & Richardson, S. S. (2014). Autism as a biomedical platform for sex differences research. *BioSocieties, 9*(3), 262–83.

CHAPTER 3. FEMALE AUTISM

1. Wood-Downie, H., Wong, B., Kovshoff, H., Cortese, S., & Hadwin, J. A. (2021). Research review: A systematic review and meta-analysis of sex/gender differences in social interaction and communication in autistic and nonautistic children and adolescents. *Journal of Child Psychology and Psychiatry, 62*(8), 922–36.

2. Achenbach, T. M., Ivanova, M. Y., Rescorla, L. A., Turner, L. V., & Althoff, R. R. (2016). Internalizing/externalizing problems: Review and recommendations for clinical and research applications. *Journal of the American Academy of Child & Adolescent Psychiatry, 55*(8), 647–56.

3. Mayes, S. D., Castagna, P. J., & Waschbusch, D. A. (2020). Sex differences in externalizing and internalizing symptoms in ADHD, autism, and

general population samples. *Journal of Psychopathology and Behavioral Assessment, 42*(3), 519–26.

4. Lundin, K., Mahdi, S., Isaksson, J., & Bölte, S. (2021). Functional gender differences in autism: An international, multidisciplinary expert survey using the International Classification of Functioning, Disability, and Health model. *Autism, 25*(4), 1020–35.

5. Grossmann, T. (2013). The role of medial prefrontal cortex in early social cognition. *Frontiers in Human Neuroscience, 7*, 340.

6. Vannasing, P., Florea, O., González-Frankenberger, B., Tremblay, J., Paquette, N., Safi, D., Wallois, F., Lepore, F., Béland, R., Lassonde, M., & Gallagher, A. (2016). Distinct hemispheric specializations for native and non-native languages in one-day-old newborns identified by fNIRS. *Neuropsychologia, 84*, 63–9.

7. Cheng, Y., Lee, S.-Y., Chen, H.-Y., Wang, P.-Y., & Decety, J. (2012). Voice and emotion processing in the human neonatal brain. *Journal of Cognitive Neuroscience, 24*(6), 1411–19.

8. Hittelman, J. H., & Dickes, R. (1979). Sex differences in neonatal eye contact time. *Merrill-Palmer Quarterly of Behavior and Development, 25*(3), 171–84.

9. Leeb, R. T., & Rejskind, F. G. (2004). Here's looking at you, kid! A longitudinal study of perceived gender differences in mutual gaze behaviour in young infants. *Sex Roles, 50*, 1–14; Smith, C., & Lloyd, B. (1978). Maternal behavior and perceived sex of infant: Revisited. *Child Development, 49*(4), 1263–5.

10. Seavey, C. A., Katz, P. A., & Zalk, S. R. (1975). Baby X: The effect of gender labels on adult responses to infants. *Sex Roles, 1*(2), 103–9; Sidorowicz, L. S., & Lunney, G. S. (1980). Baby X revisited. *Sex Roles, 6*(1), 67–73.

11. Endendijk, J. J., Groeneveld, M. G., van Berkel, S. R., Hallers-Haalboom, E. T., Mesman, J., & Bakermans-Kranenburg, M. J. (2013). Gender stereotypes in the family context: Mothers, fathers, and siblings. *Sex Roles, 68*(9–10), 577–90; Portengen, C. M., van Baar, A.L., & Endendijk, J. J. (2023). A neurocognitive approach to studying processes underlying parents' gender socialization. *Frontiers in Psychology, 13*, 1054886.

12. The Fawcett Society. (2020, December). *Unlimited potential – The final report of the commission on gender stereotypes in early childhood*. www.fawcettsociety.org.uk/unlimited-potential-the-final-report-of-the-commission-on-gender-stereotypes-in-early-childhood; LEGO Group. (2021, October 10). *Girls are ready to overcome gender norms but society continues to enforce biases that hamper their creative potential*. www.lego.com/en-us/aboutus/news/2021/september/lego-ready-for-girls-campaign; Girlguiding. Our research. www.girlguiding.org.uk/girls-making-change/our-research/.

13. Weisgram, E. S., Fulcher, M., & Dinella, L. M. (2014). Pink gives girls

permission: Exploring the roles of explicit gender labels and gender-typed colors on preschool children's toy preferences. *Journal of Applied Developmental Psychology, 35*(5), 401–9.

14. Cuff, B. M. P., Brown, S. J., Taylor, L., & Howat, D. J. (2016). Empathy: A review of the concept. *Emotion Review, 8*(2), 144–53.

15. Baron-Cohen, S. (2004). *The essential difference: Male and female brains and the truth about autism*. Penguin UK.

16. Aznar, A., & Tenenbaum, H. R. (2020). Gender comparisons in mother-child emotion talk: A meta-analysis. *Sex Roles: A Journal of Research, 82*(3–4), 155–62.

17. Greenberg, D. M., Warrier, V., Allison, C., & Baron-Cohen, S. (2018). Testing the empathizing-systemizing theory of sex differences and the extreme male brain theory of autism in half a million people. *Proceedings of the National Academy of Sciences, 115*(48), 12152–7.

18. Greenberg, D. M., Warrier, V., Abu-Akel, A., Allison, C., Gajos, K. Z., Reinecke, K., Rentfrow, P. J., Radecki, M. A., & Baron-Cohen, S. (2023). Sex and age differences in "theory of mind" across 57 countries using the English version of the "Reading the Mind in the Eyes" Test. *Proceedings of the National Academy of Sciences, 120*(1), e2022385119.

19. Kittel, A. F. D., Olderbak, S., & Wilhelm, O. (2022). Sty in the mind's eye: A meta-analytic investigation of the nomological network and internal consistency of the 'Reading the Mind in the Eyes' test. *Assessment, 29*(5), 872–95; Higgins, W. C., Ross, R. M., Langdon, R., & Polito, V. (2023). The 'Reading the Mind in the Eyes' test shows poor psychometric properties in a large, demographically representative U.S. sample. *Assessment, 30*(6), 1777–89.

20. Cheslack-Postava, K., & Jordan-Young, R. M. (2012). Autism spectrum disorders: Toward a gendered embodiment model. *Social Science & Medicine, 74*(11), 1667–74.

21. Bargiela, S., Steward, R., & Mandy, W. (2016). The experiences of late-diagnosed women with autism spectrum conditions: An investigation of the female autism phenotype. *Journal of Autism and Develomental Disorders, 46*(10), 3281–94.

22. Rivet, T. T., & Matson, J. L. (2011). Review of gender differences in core symptomatology in autism spectrum disorders. *Research in Autism Spectrum Disorders, 5*(3), 957–76.

23. Wood-Downie, H., Wong, B., Kovshoff, H., Cortese, S., & Hadwin, J. A. (2021). Research review: A systematic review and meta-analysis of sex/gender differences in social interaction and communication in autistic and nonautistic children and adolescents. *Journal of Child Psychology and Psychiatry, 62*(8), 922–36.

24. Cola, M., Yankowitz, L. D., Tena, K., Russell, A., Bateman, L., Knox, A.,

Plate, S., Cubit, L. S., Zampella, C. J., Pandey, J., Schultz, R. T., & Parish-Morris, J. (2022). Friend matters: Sex differences in social language during autism diagnostic interviews. *Molecular Autism, 13*(1), 1–16.

25. Cridland, E. K., Jones, S. C., Caputi, P., & Magee, C. A. (2014). Being a girl in a boys' world: Investigating the experiences of girls with autism spectrum disorders during adolescence. *Journal of Autism and Developmental Disorders, 44*(6), 1261–74; Tierney, S., Burns, J., & Kilbey, E. (2016). Looking behind the mask: Social coping strategies of girls on the autistic spectrum. *Research in Autism Spectrum Disorders, 23*, 73–83; Sedgewick, F., Hill, V., & Pellicano, E. (2018). Parent perspectives on autistic girls' friendships and futures. *Autism & Developmental Language Impairments, 3*, 2396941518794497.

26. Wood-Downie, H., Wong, B., Kovshoff, H., Cortese, S., & Hadwin, J. A. (2021). Research review: A systematic review and meta-analysis of sex /gender differences in social interaction and communication in autistic and nonautistic children and adolescents. *Journal of Child Psychology and Psychiatry, 62*(8), 922–36.

27. Baron-Cohen, S. (1995). *Mindblindness: An essay on autism and theory of mind*. MIT Press.

28. Kok, F. M., Groen, Y., Becke, M., Fuermaier, A. B., & Tucha, O. (2016). Self-reported empathy in adult women with autism spectrum disorders – A systematic mini review. *PLOS ONE, 11*(3), e0151568.

29. Decety, J., & Jackson, P. L. (2006). A social-neuroscience perspective on empathy. *Current Directions in Psychological Science, 15*(2), 54–5.

30. Decety, J., & Jackson, P. L. (2006). A social-neuroscience perspective on empathy. *Current Directions in Psychological Science, 15*(2), 54–5; Rieffe, C., O'Connor, R., Bülow, A., Willems, D., Hull, L., Sedgewick, F., Stockmann, L., & Blijd-Hoogewys, E. (2021). Quantity and quality of empathic responding by autistic and non-autistic adolescent girls and boys. *Autism, 25*(1), 199–209.

31. Shalev, I., Warrier, V., Greenberg, D. M., Smith, P., Allison, C., Baron-Cohen, S., Eran, A., & Uzefovsky, F. (2022). Reexamining empathy in autism: Empathic disequilibrium as a novel predictor of autism diagnosis and autistic traits. *Autism Research, 15*(10), 1917–28.

32. Sedgewick, F., Hill, V., & Pellicano, E. (2019). 'It's different for girls': Gender differences in the friendships and conflict of autistic and neurotypical adolescents. *Autism, 23*(5), 1119–32.

33. Leekam, S. R., Prior, M. R., & Uljarevic, M. (2011). Restricted and repetitive behaviors in autism spectrum disorders: A review of research in the last decade. *Psychological Bulletin, 137*(4), 562.

34. Bodfish, J. W., Symons, F. J., and Lewis, M. H. (1998). The Repetitive Behavior Scale: A test manual. Western Carolina Center Research Reports.

35. Antezana, L., Factor, R. S., Condy, E. E., Strege, M. V., Scarpa, A., &

Richey, J. A. (2019). Gender differences in restricted and repetitive behaviors and interests in youth with autism. *Autism Research, 12*(2), 274–83.

36. Nelson, S. (2022, April 6). Autism: I was diagnosed at 60. BBC. www.bbc.com/future/article/20220405-the-life-changing-diagnosis-of-autism-in-later-life.

37. Kapp, S. K., Steward, R., Crane, L., Elliott, D., Elphick, C., Pellicano, E., & Russell, G. (2019). 'People should be allowed to do what they like': Autistic adults' views and experiences of stimming. *Autism, 23*(7), 1782–92.

38. McFayden, T. C., Antezana, L., Albright, J., Muskett, A., & Scarpa, A. (2020). Sex differences in an autism spectrum disorder diagnosis: Are restricted repetitive behaviors and interests the key? *Review Journal of Autism and Developmental Disorders, 7*(2), 119–26.

39. Attwood, T. (2003). Understanding and managing circumscribed interests. In M. Prior (Ed.), *Learning and behavior problems in Asperger syndrome*. Guilford Press.

40. Tavassoli, T., Miller, L. J., Schoen, S. A., Nielsen, D. M., & Baron-Cohen, S. (2014). Sensory over-responsivity in adults with autism spectrum conditions. *Autism, 18*(4), 428–32; Kirby, A. V., Bilder, D. A., Wiggins, L. D., Hughes, M. M., Davis, J., Hall-Lande, J. A., Lee, L.-C., McMahon, W. M., & Bakian, A. V. (2022). Sensory features in autism: Findings from a large population-based surveillance system. *Autism Research, 15*(4), 751–60.

41. Osório, J. M. A., Rodríguez-Herreros, B., Richetin, S., Junod, V., Romascano, D., Pittet, V., Chabane, N., Jequier Gygax, M., & Maillard, A. M. (2021). Sex differences in sensory processing in children with autism spectrum disorder. *Autism Research, 14*(11), 2412–23.

42. Christine McGuiness (Presenter). (2023). *Unmasking my autism* [Film]. BBC One. www.bbc.co.uk/programmes/m001k31t.

43. Lockwood Estrin, G., Milner, V., Spain, D., Happé, F., & Colvert, E. (2021). Barriers to autism spectrum disorder diagnosis for young women and girls: A systematic review. *Review Journal of Autism and Developmental Disorders, 8*(4), 454–70; Taylor, E., Holt, R., Tavassoli, T., Ashwin, C., & Baron-Cohen, S. (2020). Revised scored Sensory Perception Quotient reveals sensory hypersensitivity in women with autism. *Molecular Autism, 11*(1), 1–13.

44. Kopp, S., & Gillberg, C. (2011). The Autism Spectrum Screening Questionnaire (ASSQ)–Revised Extended Version (ASSQ–REV): An instrument for better capturing the autism phenotype in girls? A preliminary study involving 191 clinical cases and community controls. *Research in Developmental Disabilities*, 32(6), 2875–88.

45. Simcoe, S. M., Brownlow, C., Garnett, M. S., Rynkiewicz, A., & Attwood, T. (2018). Profiling autism symptomatology: An exploration of the Q-ASC parental report scale in capturing sex differences in autism. *Journal of Autism and Developmental Disorders, 48*(2), 389–403.

46. Plumb, P., & Cowan, G. (1984). A developmental study of destereotyping and androgynous activity preferences of tomboys, nontomboys, and males. *Sex Roles: A Journal of Research, 10*(9–10), 703–12.

47. Clarke, E., Hull, L., Loomes, R., McCormick, C. E. B., Sheinkopf, S. J., & Mandy, W. (2021). Assessing gender differences in autism spectrum disorder using the Gendered Autism Behavioral Scale (GABS): An exploratory study. *Research in Autism Spectrum Disorders, 88*, 101844.

CHAPTER 4. BEHIND THE MASK

1. Wing, L. (1981). Sex ratios in early childhood autism and related conditions. *Psychiatry Research, 5*(2), 129–37.

2. Hull, L., Petrides, K. V., Allison, C., Smith, P., Baron-Cohen, S., Lai, M.-C., & Mandy, W. (2017). 'Putting on my best normal': Social camouflaging in adults with autism spectrum conditions. *Journal of Autism and Developmental Disorders, 47*(8), 2519–34.

3. Baker, A. R. (2002, November 10–14). *The invisible at the end of the spectrum: Shadows, residues, 'BAP', and the female Aspergers experience* [Conference presentation] Inaugural World Autism Congress: 'Unity through Diversity', Melbourne, Australia.

4. Bargiela, S., Steward, R., & Mandy, W. (2016). The experiences of late-diagnosed women with autism spectrum conditions: An investigation of the female autism phenotype. *Journal of Autism and Developmental Disorders, 46*, 3281–94; Bargiela, S. (2019). *Camouflage: The hidden lives of autistic women*. Jessica Kingsley Publishers.

5. Sedgewick, F., Hull, L., & Ellis, H. (2021). *Autism and masking: How and why people do it, and the impact it can have*. Jessica Kingsley Publishers.

6. Libsack, E. J., Keenan, E. G., Freden, C. E., Mirmina, J., Iskhakov, N., Krishnathasan, D., & Lerner, M. D. (2021). A systematic review of passing as non-autistic in autism spectrum disorder. *Clinical Child and Family Psychology Review, 24*(4), 1–30.

7. Livingston, L. A., & Happé, F. (2017). Conceptualising compensation in neurodevelopmental disorders: Reflections from autism spectrum disorder. *Neuroscience & Biobehavioral Reviews, 80*, 729–42; Livingston, L. A., Shah, P., & Happé, F. (2019). Compensatory strategies below the behavioural surface in autism: A qualitative study. *The Lancet Psychiatry, 6*(9), 766–77.

8. Belcher, H. (2022). *Taking off the mask: Practical exercises to help understand and minimise the effects of autistic camouflaging*. Jessica Kingsley Publishers.

9. Dean, M., Harwood, R., & Kasari, C. (2017). The art of camouflage: Gender differences in the social behaviors of girls and boys with autism spectrum disorder. *Autism, 21*(6), 678–89.

10. Dean, M., Harwood, R., & Kasari, C. (2017). The art of camouflage:

Gender differences in the social behaviors of girls and boys with autism spectrum disorder. *Autism, 21*(6), 678–89.

11. Milner, V., Colvert, E., Mandy, W., & Happé, F. (2023). A comparison of self-report and discrepancy measures of camouflaging: Exploring sex differences in diagnosed autistic versus high autistic trait young adults. *Autism Research, 16*(3), 580–90.

12. Lai, M.-C., Lombardo, M. V., Ruigrok, A. N. V., Chakrabarti, B., Auyeung, B., Szatmari, P., Happé, F., Baron-Cohen, S., & MRC AIMS Consortium. (2017). Quantifying and exploring camouflaging in men and women with autism. *Autism, 21*(6), 690–702.

13. Hull, L., Mandy, W., Lai, M.-C., Baron-Cohen, S., Allison, C., Smith, P., & Petrides, K. V. (2019). Development and validation of the camouflaging autistic traits questionnaire (CAT-Q). *Journal of Autism and Developmental Disorders, 49*(6), 819–33.

14. Cook, J., Hull, L., Crane, L., & Mandy, W. (2021). Camouflaging in autism: A systematic review. *Clinical Psychology Review, 89*, 02080.

15. Dunbar, R. I. M. (1993). Coevolution of neocortical size, group size and language in humans. *Behavioral and Brain Sciences, 16*(4), 681–94.

16. Baumeister, R. F., & Leary, M. R. (1995). The need to belong: Desire for interpersonal attachments as a fundamental human motivation. *Psychological Bulletin, 117*(3), 497–529.

17. Perry, E., Mandy, W., Hull, L., & Cage, E. (2022). Understanding camouflaging as a response to autism-related stigma: A social identity theory approach. *Journal of Autism and Developmental Disorders, 52*(2), 800–10.

18. Lawson, W. (2020). Adaptive morphing and coping with social threat in autism: An autistic perspective. *Journal of Intellectual Disability – Diagnosis and Treatment, 8*(8), 519–26.

19. Goffman, E. (2023). The presentation of self in everyday life. In W. Longhofer & D. Winchester (Eds.), *Social theory re-wired: New connections to classical and contemporary perspectives* (pp. 450–9). Routledge.

20. Lorenz, S., & Hull, L. (2024, January 26). Do all of us camouflage? Exploring levels of camouflaging and mental health well-being in the general population. *Trends in Psychology*, 1–15.

21. Bradley, L., Shaw, R., Baron-Cohen, S., & Cassidy, S. (2021). Autistic adults' experiences of camouflaging and its perceived impact on mental health. *Autism in Adulthood, 3*(4), 320–9.

22. Hull, L., Lai, M.-C., Baron-Cohen, S., Allison, C., Smith, P., Petrides, K. V., & Mandy, W. (2020). Gender differences in self-reported camouflaging in autistic and non-autistic adults. *Autism, 24*(2), 352–63; Milner, V., Mandy, W., Happé, F., & Colvert, E. (2023). Sex differences in predictors and outcomes of camouflaging: Comparing diagnosed autistic, high autistic trait and low autistic trait young adults. *Autism, 27*(2), 402–14.

23. Hull, L., Petrides, K. V., Allison, C., Smith, P., Baron-Cohen, S., Lai, M.-C., & Mandy, W. (2017). "Putting on my best normal": Social camouflaging in adults with autism spectrum conditions. *Journal of Autism and Developmental Disorders, 47*(8), 2519–34.

24. Cage, E., & Troxell-Whitman, Z. (2019). Understanding the reasons, contexts and costs of camouflaging for autistic adults. *Journal of Autism and Developmental Disorders, 49*(5), 1899–1911.

25. Beck, J. S., Lundwall, R. A., Gabrielsen, T., Cox, J. C., & South, M. (2020). Looking good but feeling bad: "Camouflaging" behaviors and mental health in women with autistic traits. *Autism, 24*(4), 809–21.

26. Cook, J., Hull, L., Crane, L., & Mandy, W. (2021). Camouflaging in autism: A systematic review. *Clinical Psychology Review, 89*, 102080.

27. Martini, M. I., Kuja-Halkola, R., Butwicka, A., Du Rietz, E., D'Onofrio, B. M., Happé, F., Kanina, A., Larsson, H., Lundström, S., Martin, J., Rosenqvist, M. A., Lichtenstein, P., & Taylor, M. J. (2022). Sex differences in mental health problems and psychiatric hospitalization in autistic young adults. *JAMA Psychiatry, 79*(12), 1188–98.

CHAPTER 5. THE AUTISTIC BRAIN

1. Havdahl, A., Niarchou, M., Starnawska, A., Uddin, M., van der Merwe, C., & Warrier, V. (2021). Genetic contributions to autism spectrum disorder. *Psychological Medicine, 51*(13), 2260–73; Tick, B., Bolton, P., Happé, F., Rutter, M., & Rijsdijk, F. (2016). Heritability of autism spectrum disorders: A meta-analysis of twin studies. *Journal of Child Psychology and Psychiatry, 57*(5), 585–95; Lee, B. (2020, January 7). *Autism heritability: It probably does not mean what you think it means*. The Transmitter. www.thetransmitter.org/spectrum/autism-heritability-it-probably-does-not-mean-what-you-think-it-means/.

2. Folstein, S., & Rutter, M. (1977). Genetic influences and infantile autism. *Nature, 265*, 726–8.

3. Lime Connect. (2016, March 23). *Interview with Dr. Stephen Shore: Autism advocate & on the spectrum*. International Board of Credentialing and Continuing Education Standards. https://ibcces.org/blog/2018/03/23/12748.

4. Müller, R.-A., & Fishman, I. (2018). Brain connectivity and neuroimaging of social networks in autism. *Trends in Cognitive Sciences, 22*(12), 1103–16.

5. Mitchell, K. J. (2020). *Innate: How the wiring of our brains shapes who we are*. Princeton University Press.

6. Qiu, S., Qiu, Y., Li, Y., & Cong, X. (2022). Genetics of autism spectrum disorder: An umbrella review of systematic reviews and meta-analyses. *Translational Psychiatry, 12*(1), 249; Manoli, D. S., & State, M. W. (2021). Autism spectrum disorder genetics and the search for pathological mechanisms. *American Journal of Psychiatry, 178*(1), 30–8; Zeliadt, N. (2021,

May 28). *Autism genetics, explained*. The Transmitter. www.thetransmitter.org/spectrum/autism-genetics-explained.

7. Oberman, L. M., Boccuto, L., Cascio, L., Sarasua, S., & Kaufmann, W. E. (2015). Autism spectrum disorder in Phelan-McDermid syndrome: Initial characterization and genotype-phenotype correlations. *Orphanet Journal of Rare Diseases, 10*, 1–9.

8. Lee, D. K., Li, S. W., Bounni, F., Friedman, G., Jamali, M., Strahs, L., Zeliger, O., Gabrieli, P., Stankovich, M. A., Demaree, J., & Williams, Z. M. (2021). Reduced sociability and social agency encoding in adult Shank3-mutant mice are restored through gene re-expression in real time. *Nature Neuroscience, 24*(9), 1243–55.

9. Havdahl, A., Niarchou, M., Starnawska, A., Uddin, M., van der Merwe, C., & Warrier, V. (2021). Genetic contributions to autism spectrum disorder. *Psychological Medicine, 51*(13), 2260–73.

10. Nisar, S., & Haris, M. (2023). Neuroimaging genetics approaches to identify new biomarkers for the early diagnosis of autism spectrum disorder. *Molecular Psychiatry, 28*, 4995–5008.

11. SFRI Gene. https://gene.sfari.org.

12. Wigdor, E. M., Weiner, D. J., Grove, J., Fu, J. M., Thompson, W. K., Carey, C. E., Baya, N., van der Merwe, C., Walters, R. K., Satterstrom, F. K., Palmer, D. S., et al. (2022). The female protective effect against autism spectrum disorder. *Cell Genomics, 2*(6), 100134.

13. Marco, E. J., & Skuse, D. H. (2006). Autism-lessons from the X chromosome. *Social Cognitive and Affective Neuroscience, 1*(3), 183–93; Brand, B. A., Blesson, A. E., & Smith-Hicks, C. L. (2021). The impact of X-chromosome inactivation on phenotypic expression of X-linked neurodevelopmental disorders. *Brain Sciences, 11*(7), 904.

14. Nguyen, T. A., Lehr, A. W., and Roche, K. W. (2020). Neuroligins and neurodevelopmental disorders: X-linked genetics. *Frontiers in Synaptic Neuroscience, 12*, 33.

15. Aishworiya, R., Protic, D., & Hagerman, R. (2022). Autism spectrum disorder in the fragile X premutation state: Possible mechanisms and implications. *Journal of Neurology, 269*(9), 4676–83.

16. Robinson, E. B., Lichtenstein, P., Anckarsäter, H., Happé, F., & Ronald, A. (2013). Examining and interpreting the female protective effect against autistic behavior. *Proceedings of the National Academy of Sciences, 110*(13), 5258–62; Zhang, Y., Li, N., Li, C., Zhang, Z., Teng, H., Wang, Y., Zhao, T., Shi, L., Zhang, K., Xia, K., Li, J., & Sun, Z. (2020). Genetic evidence of gender difference in autism spectrum disorder supports the female-protective effect. *Translational Psychiatry, 10*(1), 4.

17. Elsabbagh, M., & Johnson, M. H. (2016). Autism and the social brain: The first-year puzzle. *Biological Psychiatry, 80*(2), 94–9.

18. Dr. Lila Landowski. (2021, November 14). *Finding that connection* [Video]. YouTube. www.youtube.com/watch?v=Rvmvt7gscIM.

19. Connectome Coordination Facility. www.humanconnectome.org.

20. Courchesne, E., Pierce, K., Schumann, C. M., Redcay, E., Buckwalter, J. A., Kennedy, D. P., & Morgan, J. (2007). Mapping early brain development in autism. *Neuron, 56*(2), 99–413.

21. Messinger, D., Young, G. S., Ozonoff, S., Dobkins, K., Carter, A., Zwaigenbaum, L., Landa, R. J., Charman, T., Stone, W. L., Constantino, J. N., Hutman, T., et al. (2013). Beyond autism: A baby siblings research consortium study of high-risk children at three years of age. *Journal of the American Academy of Child and Adolescent Psychiatry, 52*(3), 300–8; Szatmari, P., Chawarska, K., Dawson, G., Georgiades, S., Landa, R., Lord, C., Messinger, D. S., Thurm, A., & Halladay, A. (2016). Prospective longitudinal studies of infant siblings of children with autism: Lessons learned and future directions. *Journal of the American Academy of Child and Adolescent Psychiatry, 55*(3), 179–87.

22. Lee, J. K., Andrews, D. S., Ozonoff, S., Solomon, M., Rogers, S., Amaral, D. G., & Nordahl, C. W. (2021). Longitudinal evaluation of cerebral growth across childhood in boys and girls with autism spectrum disorder. *Biological Psychiatry, 90*(5), 286–94.

23. Lewis, J. D., Evans, A. C., Pruett, J. R., Botteron, K., Zwaigenbaum, L., Estes, A., Gerig, G., Collins, L., Kostopoulos, P., McKinstry, R., Dager, S., et al. (2014). Network inefficiencies in autism spectrum disorder at 24 months. *Translational Psychiatry, 4*(5), e388.

24. Ciarrusta, J., Dimitrova, R., Batalle, D., O'Muircheartaigh, J., Cordero-Grande, L., Price, A., Hughes, E., et al. (2020). Emerging functional connectivity differences in newborn infants vulnerable to autism spectrum disorders. *Translational Psychiatry, 10*, 131.

25. Wang, S., & Li, X. (2023). A revisit of the amygdala theory of autism: Twenty years after. *Neuropsychologia, 183*, 108519.

26. Rippon, G. (2024). Differently different? A commentary on the emerging social cognitive neuroscience of female autism. *Biology of Sex Differences, 15*(1), 49.

27. Mo, K., Sadoway, T., Bonato, S., Ameis, S. H., Anagnostou, E., Lerch, J. P., Taylor, M. J., & Lai, M.-C. (2021). Sex/gender differences in the human autistic brains: A systematic review of 20 years of neuroimaging research. *NeuroImage: Clinical, 32*, 102811.

28. Lai, M.-C., Lombardo, M. V., Auyeung, B., Chakrabarti, B., & Baron-Cohen, S. (2015). Sex/gender differences and autism: Setting the scene for future research. *Journal of the American Academy of Child and Adolescent Psychiatry, 54*(1), 11–24.

29. Schumann, C. M., Bloss, C. S., Barnes, C. C., Wideman, G. M., Carper, R. A., Akshoomoff, N., Pierce, K., Hagler, D., Schork, N., Lord, C., & Courchesne, E. (2010). Longitudinal magnetic resonance imaging study of

cortical development through early childhood in autism. *Journal of Neuroscience, 30*(12), 4419–27.

30. Cauvet, É., Van't Westeinde, A., Toro, R., Kuja-Halkola, R., Neufeld, J., Mevel, K., & Bölte, S. (2020). The social brain in female autism: A structural imaging study of twins. *Social Cognitive and Affective Neuroscience, 15*(4), 423–36.

31. Hernandez, L. M., Lawrence, K. E., Padgaonkar, N. T., Inada, M., Hoekstra, J. N., Lowe, J. K., Eilbott, J., Jack, A., Aylward, E., Gaab, N., Van Horn, J. D., et al. (2020). Imaging-genetics of sex differences in ASD: Distinct effects of *OXTR* variants on brain connectivity. *Translational Psychiatry, 10*(1), 82.

32. Lawrence, K. E., Hernandez, L. M., Fuster, E., Padgaonkar, N. T., Patterson, G., Jung, J., Okada, N. J., Lowe, J. K., Hoekstra, J. N., Jack, A., Aylward, E., et al. (2022). Impact of autism genetic risk on brain connectivity: A mechanism for the female protective effect. *Brain, 145*(1), 378–87.

CHAPTER 6. ON BEING SOCIAL

1. Kanner, L. (1943). Autistic disturbances of affective contact. *Nervous Child, 2*, 217–50.

2. Lockwood, P. L., Apps, M.A. J., & Chang, S. W. C. (2020). Is there a 'social' brain? Implementations and algorithms. *Trends in Cognitive Sciences, 24*(10), 802–13; Arioli, M., Gianelli, C., & Canessa, N. (2021). Neural representation of social concepts: A coordinate-based meta-analysis of fMRI studies. *Brain Imaging and Behavior, 15*(4), 1912–21.

3. Mundy, P., & Newell, L. (2007). Attention, joint attention, and social cognition. *Current Directions in Psychological Science, 16*(5), 269–74; Constantino, J. N., Kennon-McGill, S., Weichselbaum, C., Marrus, N., Haider, A., Glowinski, A. L., Gillespie, S., Klaiman, C., Klin, A., & Jones, W. (2017). Infant viewing of social scenes is under genetic control and is atypical in autism. *Nature, 547*(7663), 340–4.

4. Lombardo, M. V., Chakrabarti, B., Bullmore, E. T., Sadek, S. A., Pasco, G., Wheelwright, S. J., Suckling, J., MRC AIMS Consortium, & Baron-Cohen, S. (2010). Atypical neural self-representation in autism. *Brain, 133*(2), 611–24.

5. Frith, C. D. (2007). The social brain? *Philosophical Transactions of the Royal Society B: Biological Sciences, 362*(1480), 671–8; Adolphs, R. (2009). The social brain: neural basis of social knowledge. *Annual Review of Psychology, 60*, 693–716.

6. Dalgleish, T., Walsh, N. D., Mobbs, D., Schweizer, S., van Harmelen, A.-L., Dunn, B., Dunn, V., Goodyer, I., & Stretton, J. (2017). Social pain and social gain in the adolescent brain: A common neural circuitry underlying both positive and negative social evaluation. *Scientific Reports, 7*(1), 42010.

7. Eisenberger, N. I. (2015). Social pain and the brain: Controversies, questions, and where to go from here. *Annual Review of Psychology, 66*(1), 601–29.

8. Pfeiffer, U. J., Schilbach, L., Timmermans, B., Kuzmanovic, B., Georgescu, A. L., Bente, G., & Vogeley, K. (2014). Why we interact: On the functional role of the striatum in the subjective experience of social interaction. *NeuroImage, 101*, 124–37; Rilling, J. K., & Sanfey, A. G. (2011). The neuroscience of social decision-making. *Annual Review of Psychology, 62*(1), 23–48.

9. Dichter, G. S., Felder, J. N., Bodfish, J. W., Sikich, L., & Belger, A. (2009). Mapping social target detection with functional magnetic resonance imaging. *Social Cognitive and Affective Neuroscience, 4*(1), 59–69.

10. Somerville, L. H., Hare, T., & Casey, B. J. (2011). Frontostriatal maturation predicts cognitive control failure to appetitive cues in adolescents. *Journal of Cognitive Neuroscience, 23*(9), 2123–34.

11. Schaafsma, S. M., Pfaff, D. W., Spunt, R. P., & Adolphs, R. (2015). Deconstructing and reconstructing theory of mind. *Trends in Cognitive Sciences, 19*(2), 65–72.

12. Wimmer, H., & Perner, J. (1983). Beliefs about beliefs: Representation and constraining function of wrong beliefs in young children's understanding of deception. *Cognition, 13*(1), 103–28.

13. Baron-Cohen, S., Leslie, A. M., & Frith, U. (1985). Does the autistic child have a "theory of mind"? *Cognition, 21*(1), 37–46; Baron-Cohen, S. (2000). Theory of mind and autism: A review. *International Review of Research in Mental Retardation, 23*, 169–84; Gallagher, H. L., & Frith, C. D. (2003). Functional imaging of 'theory of mind'. *Trends in Cognitive Sciences, 7*(2), 77–83; Schurz, M., Radua, J., Aichhorn, M., Richlan, F., & Perner, J. (2014). Fractionating theory of mind: A meta-analysis of functional brain imaging studies. *Neuroscience and Biobehavioral Reviews, 42*, 9–34.

14. Baron-Cohen, S., Leslie, A. M., & Frith, U. (1985). Does the autistic child have a "theory of mind"? *Cognition, 21*(1), 37–46; Baron-Cohen, S. (2000). Theory of mind and autism: A review. *International Review of Research in Mental Retardation, 23*, 169–84; Gallagher, H. L., & Frith, C. D. (2003). Functional imaging of 'theory of mind'. *Trends in Cognitive Sciences, 7*(2), 77–83; Schurz, M., Radua, J., Aichhorn, M., Richlan, F., & Perner, J. (2014). Fractionating theory of mind: A meta-analysis of functional brain imaging studies. *Neuroscience and Biobehavioral Reviews, 42*, 9–34.

15. Arioli, M., Gianelli, C., & Canessa, N. (2021). Neural representation of social concepts: A coordinate-based meta-analysis of fMRI studies. *Brain Imaging and Behavior, 15*(4), 1912–21.

16. Ochsner, K. N., Ray, R. D., Cooper, J. C., Robertson, E. R., Chopra, S., Gabrieli, J. D., & Gross, J. J. (2004). For better or for worse: Neural systems supporting the cognitive down- and up-regulation of negative emotion. *Neuroimage, 23*(2), 483–99.

17. Apps, M. A., Rushworth, M. F. S., & Chang, S. W. C. (2016). The anterior cingulate gyrus and social cognition: Tracking the motivation of others. *Neuron, 90*(4), 692–707.

18. Gotts, S. J., Simmons, W. K., Milbury, L. A., Wallace, G. L., Cox, R. W., & Martin, A. (2012). Fractionation of social brain circuits in autism spectrum disorders. *Brain, 135*(9), 2711–25.

19. von dem Hagen, E. A. H., Stoyanova, R. S., Baron-Cohen, S., & Calder, A. J. (2013). Reduced functional connectivity within and between 'social' resting state networks in autism spectrum conditions. *Social Cognitive and Affective Neuroscience, 8*(6), 694–701.

20. Marshall, E., Nomi, J. S., Dirks, B., Romero, C., Kupis, L., Chang, C., & Uddin, L. Q. (2020). Coactivation pattern analysis reveals altered salience network dynamics in children with autism spectrum disorder. *Network Neuroscience, 4*(4), 1219–34.

21. Friston, K. (2010). The free-energy principle: A unified brain theory? *Nature Reviews Neuroscience, 11*, 127–138; Friston, K. J., Stephan, K. E., Montague, R., & Dolan, R. J. (2014). Computational psychiatry: The brain as a phantastic organ. *The Lancet Psychiatry, 1*(2), 148–58.

22. Pellicano, E., & Burr, D. (2012). When the world becomes 'too real': A Bayesian explanation of autistic perception. *Trends in Cognitive Sciences, 16*(10), 504–10; Friston, K. J., Lawson, R., & Frith, C. D. (2013). On hyperpriors and hypopriors: Comment on Pellicano and Burr. *Trends in Cognitive Sciences, 17*(1), 1; Lawson, R. P., Rees, G., & Friston, K. J. (2014). An aberrant precision account of autism. *Frontiers in Human Neuroscience, 8*, 302.

23. Kessler, K., Seymour, R. A., & Rippon, G. (2016). Brain oscillations and connectivity in autism spectrum disorders (ASD): New approaches to methodology, measurement and modelling. *Neuroscience and Biobehavioral Reviews, 71*, 601–20.

24. Seymour, R. A., Rippon, G., & Kessler, K. (2017). The detection of phase amplitude coupling during sensory processing. *Frontiers in Neuroscience, 11*, 487.

25. Seymour, R. A., Rippon, G., Gooding-Williams, G., Schoffelen, J. M., & Kessler, K. (2019). Dysregulated oscillatory connectivity in the visual system in autism spectrum disorder. *Brain, 142*(10), 3294–3305.

26. Van de Cruys, S., Evers, K., Van der Hallen, R., Van Eylen, L., Boets, B., de-Wit, L., & Wagemans, J. (2014). Precise minds in uncertain worlds: Predictive coding in autism. *Psychological Review, 121*(4), 649.

27. Brown, E. C., & Brüne, M. (2012). The role of prediction in social neuroscience. *Frontiers in Human Neuroscience, 6*, 147.

CHAPTER 7. KANNER BRAINS AND CHAMELEON BRAINS

1. American Psychiatric Association. (2013). *Diagnostic and statistical manual of mental disorders, fifth edition: DSM-5*. American Psychiatric Association.

2. Eliot, L., Ahmed, A., Khan, H., & Patel, J. (2021). Dump the "dimorphism": Comprehensive synthesis of human brain studies reveals few male-female differences beyond size. *Neuroscience & Biobehavioral Reviews, 125*, 667–97.

3. Greenberg, D. M., Warrier, V., Abu-Akel, A., Allison, C., Gajos, K. Z., Reinecke, K., Rentfrow, P. J., Radecki, M. A., & Baron-Cohen, S. (2023). Sex and age differences in "theory of mind" across 57 countries using the English version of the "Reading the Mind in the Eyes" Test. *Proceedings of the National Academy of Sciences, 120*(1), e2022385119.

4. Mo, K., Sadoway, T., Bonato, S., Ameis, S. H., Anagnostou, E., Lerch, J. P., Taylor, M. J., & Lai, M.-C. (2021). Sex/gender differences in the human autistic brains: A systematic review of 20 years of neuroimaging research. *NeuroImage: Clinical,* 32, 102811.

5. Lombardo, M. V., Lai, M.-C., & Baron-Cohen, S. (2019). Big data approaches to decomposing heterogeneity across the autism spectrum. *Molecular Psychiatry,* 24(10), 1435–50.

6. Di Martino, A., Yan, C.-G., Li, Q., Denio, E., Castellanos, F. X., Alaerts, K., Anderson, J. S., Assaf, M., Bookheimer, S. Y., Dapretto, M., Deen, B., et al. (2014). The autism brain imaging data exchange: Towards a large-scale evaluation of the intrinsic brain architecture in autism. *Molecular Psychiatry, 19*(6), 659–67.

7. Di Martino, A., O'Connor, D., Chen, B., Alaerts, K., Anderson, J. S., Assaf, M., Balsters, J. H., Baxter, L., Beggiato, A., Bernaerts, S., Blanken, L. M. E., et al. (2017). Enhancing studies of the connectome in autism using the autism brain imaging data exchange II. *Scientific Data, 4*(1), 1–15.

8. Feliciano, P., Daniels, A. M., Snyder, L. G., Beaumont, A., Camba, A., Esler, A., Gulsrud, A. G., Mason, A., Gutierrez, A., Nicholson, A., & Paolicelli, A. M. (2018). SPARK: A US cohort of 50,000 families to accelerate autism research. *Neuron, 97*(3), 488–93.

9. Loth, E., Charman, T., Mason, L., Tillmann, J., Jones, E. J. H., Wooldridge, C., Ahmad, J., Auyeung, B., Brogna, C., Ambrosino, S., Banaschewski, T., et al. (2017). The EU-AIMS Longitudinal European Autism Project (LEAP): Design and methodologies to identify and validate stratification biomarkers for autism spectrum disorders. *Molecular Autism, 8*(1), 1–19.

10. D'Mello, A. M., Frosch, I. R., Li, C. E., Cardinaux, A. L., & Gabrieli, J. D. (2022). Exclusion of females in autism research: Empirical evidence for a 'leaky' recruitment-to-research pipeline. *Autism Research, 15*(10), 1929–40.

11. Janouschek, H., Chase, H. W., Sharkey, R. J., Peterson, Z. J., Camilleri, J. A., Abel, T., Eickhoff, S. B., & Nickl-Jockschat, T. (2021). The functional neural architecture of dysfunctional reward processing in autism. *NeuroImage: Clinical, 31,* 102700.

12. Di Martino, A., Ross, K., Uddin, L. Q., Sklar, A. B., Castellanos, F. X., & Milham, M. P. (2009). Functional brain correlates of social and nonsocial processes in autism spectrum disorders: An activation likelihood estimation meta-analysis. *Biological Psychiatry,* 65(1), 63–74; Dickstein, D. P., Pescosolido, M. F., Reidy, B. L., Galvan, T., Kim, K. L., Seymour, K. E., Laird, A. R.,

Di Martino, A., & Barrett, R. P. (2013). Developmental meta-analysis of the functional neural correlates of autism spectrum disorders. *Journal of the American Academy of Child and Adolescent Psychiatry*, 52(3), 279–89; Patriquin, M. A., DeRamus, T., Libero, L. E., Laird, A., & Kana, R. K. (2016). Neuroanatomical and neurofunctional markers of social cognition in autism spectrum disorder. *Human Brain Mapping*, 37(11), 3957–78; Clements, C. C., Zoltowski, A. R., Yankowitz, L. D., Yerys, B. E., Schultz, R. T., & Herrington, J. D. (2018). Evaluation of the social motivation hypothesis of autism: A systematic review and meta-analysis. *JAMA Psychiatry*, 75(8), 797–808; Bottini, S. (2018). Social reward processing in individuals with autism spectrum disorder: A systematic review of the social motivation hypothesis. *Research in Autism Spectrum Disorders*, 45, 9–26; Nair, A., Jolliffe, M., Lograsso, Y. S. S., & Bearden, C. E. (2020). A review of default mode network connectivity and its association with social cognition in adolescents with autism spectrum disorder and early-onset psychosis. *Frontiers in Psychiatry*, 11, 614.

13. Rippon, G. (2024). Differently different? A commentary on the emerging social cognitive neuroscience of female autism. *Biology of Sex Differences*, 15(1), 49.

14. Gender Exploration of Neurogenetics and Development to Advanced Autism Research (GENDAAR 2.0). https://psychiatry.uw.edu/project/gender-exploration-of-neurogenetics-and-development-to-advanced-autism-research-gendaar-2-0.

15. Scott-Van Zeeland, A. A., Dapretto, M., Ghahremani, D. G., Poldrack, R. A., & Bookheimer, S. Y. (2010). Reward processing in autism. *Autism Research*, 3(2), 53–67.

16. Lawrence, K. E., Hernandez, L. M., Eilbott, J., Jack, A., Aylward, E., Gaab, N., Van Horn, J. D., Bernier, R. A., Geschwind, D. H., McPartland, J. C., Nelson, C.A., et al. (2020). Neural responsivity to social rewards in autistic female youth. *Translational Psychiatry*, 10(1), 178.

17. Green, S. A., Hernandez, L., Tottenham, N., Krasileva, K., Bookheimer, S. Y., & Dapretto, M. (2015). Neurobiology of sensory overresponsivity in youth with autism spectrum disorders. *JAMA Psychiatry*, 72(8), 778–86.

18. Cummings, K. K., Lawrence, K. E., Hernandez, L. M., Wood, E. T., Bookheimer, S. Y., Dapretto, M., & Green, S. A. (2020). Sex differences in salience network connectivity and its relationship to sensory over-responsivity in youth with autism spectrum disorder. *Autism Research*, 13(9), 1489–1500.

19. Hull, J. V., Dokovna, L. B., Jacokes, Z. J., Torgerson, C. M., Irimia, A., & Van Horn, J. D. (2017). Resting-state functional connectivity in autism spectrum disorders: A review. *Frontiers in Psychiatry*, 7, 205.

20. Lawrence, K. E., Hernandez, L. M., Bowman, H. C., Padgaonkar, N. T., Fuster, E., Jack, A., Aylward, E., Gaab, N., Van Horn, J. D., Bernier,

R. A., Geschwind, D. H., et al. (2020). Sex differences in functional connectivity of the salience, default mode, and central executive networks in youth with ASD. *Cerebral Cortex, 30*(9), 5107–20.

21. Lai, M.-C., Lombardo, M. V., Chakrabarti, B., Ruigrok, A. N. V., Bullmore, E. T., Suckling, J., Auyeung, B., Happé, F., Szatmari, P., & Baron-Cohen, S. (2019). Neural self-representation in autistic women and association with 'compensatory camouflaging'. *Autism, 23*(5), 1210–23.

22. Lai, M.-C., Lombardo, M. V., Chakrabarti, B., Ruigrok, A. N. V., Bullmore, E. T., Suckling, J., Auyeung, B., Happé, F., Szatmari, P., & Baron-Cohen, S. (2019). Neural self-representation in autistic women and association with 'compensatory camouflaging'. *Autism, 23*(5), 1210–23.

23. Walsh, M. J. M., Pagni, B., Monahan, L., Delaney, S., Smith, C. J., Baxter, L., & Braden, B. B. (2022). Sex-related brain connectivity correlates of compensation in adults with autism: Insights into female protection. *Cerebral Cortex, 33*(2), 316–29.

24. Vuilleumier, P., Armony, J. L., Driver, J., & Dolan, R. J. (2003). Distinct spatial frequency sensitivities for processing faces and emotional expressions. *Nature Neuroscience, 6*(6), 624–31.

25. Lacroix, A., Harquel, S., Mermillod, M., Garrido, M., Barbosa, L., Vercueil, L., Aleysson, D., Dutheil, F., Kovarski, K., & Gomot, M. (2024). Sex modulation of faces prediction error in the autistic brain. *Communications Biology, 7*(1), 127.

26. Pang, C. (2020). *Explaining humans: What science can teach us about life, love and relationships*. Viking.

CHAPTER 8. FEMALE, AUTISTIC, AND ADOLESCENT

1. Anti-Bullying Alliance. *Prevalance of bullying*. https://anti-bullyingalliance.org.uk/tools-information/all-about-bullying/prevalence-and-impact-bullying/prevalence-bullying; U.S. Department of Health and Human Services. *Facts about bullying*. www.stopbullying.gov/resources/facts#:~:text=How%20Common%20Is%20Bullying,perception%20of%20them%20(56%25); Vogels, E. A. (2022, December 15). *Teens and cyberbullying 2022*. Pew Research Center. www.pewresearch.org/internet/2022/12/15/teens-and-cyberbullying-2022; UNESCO. (2020, November 3). *What you need to know about school violence and bullying*. www.unesco.org/en/articles/what-you-need-know-about-school-violence-and-bullying.

2. Greenlee, J. L., Winter, M. A., & Marcovici, I. A. (2020). Brief report: Gender differences in experiences of peer victimization among adolescents with autism spectrum disorder. *Journal of Autism and Developmental Disorders, 50*(10), 3790–9.

3. World Health Organization. World Mental Health Day 2021. Key messages. www.who.int/key-messages; NHS England. (2020, October 22).

Mental health of children and young people in England, 2020: Wave 1 follow up to the 2017 survey. https://digital.nhs.uk/data-and-information/publications/statistical/mental-health-of-children-and-young-people-in-england/2020-wave-1-follow-up; NHS England. (2023, November 21). *One in five children and young people had a probable mental disorder in 2023.* www.england.nhs.uk/2023/11/one-in-five-children-and-young-people-had-a-probable-mental-disorder-in-2023; U.S. Centers for Disease Control and Prevention. Youth Risk Behavior Surveillance System (YRBSS). U.S. Department of Health & Human Services. www.cdc.gov/healthyyouth/data/yrbs/index.htm; U.S. Centers for Disease Control and Prevention. (Updated 2024, May 2). *Adolescent and school health.* U.S. Department of Health & Human Services. www.cdc.gov/healthyyouth/mental-health/mental-health-numbers.html; U.S. Centers for Disease Control and Prevention. (2023, February 13). *U.S. teen girls experiencing increased sadness and violence.* U.S. Department of Health & Human Services. www.cdc.gov/media/releases/2023/p0213-yrbs.html.

4. Lai, M.-C., Kassee, C., Besney, R., Bonato, S., Hull, L., Mandy, W., Szatmari, P., & Ameis, S. H. (2019). Prevalence of co-occurring mental health diagnoses in the autism population: A systematic review and meta-analysis. *The Lancet Psychiatry, 6*(10), 819–29.

5. Vasa, R. A., & Mazurek, M. O. (2015). An update on anxiety in youth with autism spectrum disorders. *Current Opinion in Psychiatry, 28*(2), 83–90; Thiele-Swift, H. N., & Dorstyn, D.-S. (2024). Anxiety prevalence in youth with autism: A systematic review and meta-analysis of methodological and sample moderators. *Review Journal of Autism and Developmental Disorders*, 1–14; Hudson, C. C., Hall, L., & Harkness, K. L. (2019). Prevalence of depressive disorders in individuals with autism spectrum disorder: A meta-analysis. *Journal of Abnormal Child Psychology, 47*(1), 165–75.

6. Martini, M. I., Kuja-Halkola, R., Butwicka, A., Du Rietz, E., D'Onofrio, B. M., Happé, F., Kanina, A., Larsson, H., Lundström, S., Martin, J., Rosenqvist, M. A., Lichtenstein, P., & Taylor, M. J. (2022). Sex differences in mental health problems and psychiatric hospitalization in autistic young adults. *JAMA Psychiatry, 79*(12), 1188–98; Sedgewick, F., Leppanen, J., & Tchanturia, K. (2020). Gender differences in mental health prevalence in autism. *Advances in Autism, 7*(3), 208–24.

7. Picci, G., & Scherf, K. S. (2015). A two-hit model of autism: Adolescence as the second hit. *Clinical Psychological Science, 3*(3), 349–71.

8. Picci, G., & Scherf, K. S. (2015). A two-hit model of autism: Adolescence as the second hit. *Clinical Psychological Science, 3*(3), 349–71.

9. Mandy, W., Pellicano, L., St. Pourcain, B., Skuse, D., & Heron, J. (2018). The development of autistic social traits across childhood and adolescence in males and females. *Journal of Child Psychology and Psychiatry, 59*(11), 1143–51.

10. Ferri, S. L., Abel, T., & Brodkin, E. S. (2018). Sex differences in autism spectrum disorder: A review. *Current Psychiatry Reports, 20*(2), 1–17.

11. James, L. (2017). *Odd girl out: An autistic woman in a neurotypical world.* Seal Press.

12. Westwood, H., & Tchanturia, K. (2017). Autism spectrum disorder in anorexia nervosa: An updated literature review. *Current Psychiatry Reports, 19*(7), 1–10.

13. Cook, J., Hull, L., & Mandy, W. (2024). Improving diagnostic procedures in autism for girls and women: A narrative review. *Neuropsychiatric Disease and Treatment, 20*, 505–14.

14. Giedd, J. N., Blumenthal, J., Jeffries, N. O., Castellanos, F. X., Liu, H., Zijdenbos, A., Paus, T., Evans, A. C., & Rapoport, J. L. (1999). Brain development during childhood and adolescence: A longitudinal MRI study. *Nature Neuroscience,* 2(10), 861–3; Giedd, J. N. (2004). Structural magnetic resonance imaging of the adolescent brain. *Annals of the New York Academy of Sciences, 1021*(1), 77–85.

15. Váša, F., Romero-Garcia, R., Kitzbichler, M. G., Seidlitz, J., Whitaker, K. J., Vaghi, M. M., Kundu, P., Patel, A. X., Fonagy, P., Dolan, R. J., Jones, P. B., et al. (2020). Conservative and disruptive modes of adolescent change in human brain functional connectivity. *Proceedings of the National Academy of Sciences, 117*(6), 3248–53.

16. Fan, F., Liao, X., Lei, T., Zhao, T., Xia, M., Men, W., Wang, Y., Hu, M., Liu, J., Qin, S., Tan, S., et al. (2021). Development of the default-mode network during childhood and adolescence: A longitudinal resting-state fMRI study. *NeuroImage, 226*, 117581.

17. Long, E. U., Wheeler, N. E., & Cunningham, W. A. (2020). Through the looking glass: Distinguishing neural correlates of relational and nonrelational self-reference and person representation. *Cortex, 130*, 257–74.

18. Somerville, L. H., Hare, T., & Casey, B. J. (2011). Frontostriatal maturation predicts cognitive control failure to appetitive cues in adolescents. *Journal of Cognitive Neuroscience, 23*(9), 2123–34.

19. Insel, C., Kastman, E. K., Glenn, C. R., & Somerville, L. H. (2017). Development of corticostriatal connectivity constrains goal-directed behavior during adolescence. *Nature Communications, 8*(1), 1605.

20. Grosbras, M.-H., Jansen, M., Leonard, G., McIntosh, A., Osswald, K., Poulsen, C., Steinberg, L., Toro, R., & Paus, T. (2007). Neural mechanisms of resistance to peer influence in early adolescence. *Journal of Neuroscience, 27*(30), 8040–5.

21. Guyer, A. E., McClure-Tone, E. B., Shiffrin, N. D., Pine, D. S., & Nelson, E. E. (2009). Probing the neural correlates of anticipated peer evaluation in adolescence. *Child Development, 80*(4), 1000–15.

22. Zimmer-Gembeck, M. J., Gardner, A. A., Hawes, T., Masters, M. R., Waters, A. M., & Farrell, L. J. (2021). Rejection sensitivity and the development of social anxiety symptoms during adolescence: A five-year longitudinal study. *International Journal of Behavioral Development, 45*(3), 204–15; Troop-Gordon, W. (2017). Peer victimization in adolescence: The nature, progression, and consequences of being bullied within a developmental context. *Journal of Adolescence, 55*, 116–28.

23. Williams, K. D., Cheung, C. K., & Choi, W. (2000). Cyberostracism: Effects of being ignored over the Internet. *Journal of Personality and Social Psychology, 79*(5), 748.

24. Masten, C. L., Eisenberger, N. I., Borofsky, L. A., Pfeifer, J. H., McNealy, K., Mazziotta, J. C., & Dapretto, M. (2009). Neural correlates of social exclusion during adolescence: Understanding the distress of peer rejection. *Social Cognitive and Affective Neuroscience, 4*(2), 143–57.

25. Kiefer, M., Sim, E.-J., Heil, S., Brown, R., Herrnberger, B., Spitzer, M., & Grön, G. (2021). Neural signatures of bullying experience and social rejection in teenagers. *PLOS ONE, 16*(8), e0255681.

26. Lawrence, K. E., Hernandez, L. M., Bookheimer, S. Y., & Dapretto, M. (2019). Atypical longitudinal development of functional connectivity in adolescents with autism spectrum disorder. *Autism Research, 12*(1), 53–65.

27. Masten, C. L., Colich, N. L., Rudie, J. D., Bookheimer, S. Y., Eisenberger, N. I., & Dapretto, M. (2011). An fMRI investigation of responses to peer rejection in adolescents with autism spectrum disorders. *Developmental Cognitive Neuroscience, 1*(3), 260–70.

28. Lawrence, K. E., Hernandez, L. M., Eilbott, J., Jack, A., Aylward, E., Gaab, N., Van Horn, J. D., Bernier, R. A., Geschwind, D. H., McPartland, J. C., Nelson, C. A., et al. (2020). Neural responsivity to social rewards in autistic female youth. *Translational Psychiatry, 10*(1), 178.

29. Horwitz, E., Vos, M., De Bildt, A., Greaves-Lord, K., Rommelse, N., Schoevers, R., & Hartman, C. (2023). Sex differences in the course of autistic and co-occurring psychopathological symptoms in adolescents with and without autism spectrum disorder. *Autism, 27*(6), 1716–29.

30. Neustatter, A. (2015, July 14). 'Autism is seen as a male thing – but girls just implode emotionally'. *The Guardian*. www.theguardian.com/education/2015/jul/14/autism-girls-emotion-self-harm-school.

31. National Institute of Mental Health. *Eating Disorders*. (Last reviewed 2024, January). U.S. Department of Health and Human Services. www.nimh.nih.gov/health/topics/eating-disorders; National Health Service. (Last reviewed 2024, January 23). *Overview – Eating disorders*. www.nhs.uk/mental-health/feelings-symptoms-behaviours/behaviours/eating-disorders/overview/.

32. van Eeden, A. E., van Hoeken, D., & Hoek, H. W. (2021). Incidence,

prevalence and mortality of anorexia nervosa and bulimia nervosa. *Current Opinion in Psychiatry, 34*(6), 515–24.

33. Gillberg, C. (1983). Are autism and anorexia nervosa related? *British Journal of Psychiatry, 142*(4), 428; Gillberg, C. (1985). Autism and anorexia nervosa: Related conditions? *Nordisk Psykiatrisk Tidsskrift, 39*(4), 307–12.

34. Dattaro, L. (2020, December 7). *Anorexia's link to autism, explained.* The Transmitter. www.thetransmitter.org/spectrum/anorexias-link-to-autism-explained; Westwood, H., & Tchanturia, K. (2017). Autism spectrum disorder in anorexia nervosa: An updated literature review. *Current Psychiatry Reports, 19*(7), 41.

35. Mayes, S. D., & Zickgraf, H. (2019). Atypical eating behaviors in children and adolescents with autism, ADHD, other disorders, and typical development. *Research in Autism Spectrum Disorders, 64*, 76–83.

36. Adams, K. L., Mandy, W., Catmur, C., & Bird, G. (2024). Potential mechanisms underlying the association between feeding and eating disorders and autism. *Neuroscience & Biobehavioral Reviews, 162*, 105717.

37. Boltri, M., & Sapuppo, W. (2021). Anorexia nervosa and autism spectrum disorder: A systematic review. *Psychiatry Research, 306*, 114271.

38. Freeman, H. (2023). *Good girls: A story and study of anorexia.* Simon and Schuster.

39. The Emily Program. (2020, April 28). *Who am I without my eating disorder?* https://emilyprogram.com/blog/who-am-i-without-my-eating-disorder.

40. Brede, J., Babb, C., Jones, C., Elliott, M., Zanker, C., Tchanturia, K., Serpell, L., Fox, J., & Mandy, W. (2020). 'For me, the anorexia is just a symptom, and the cause is the autism': Investigating restrictive eating disorders in autistic women. *Journal of Autism and Developmental Disorders, 50*(12), 4280–96.

41. Christine McGuiness (Presenter). (2023). *Unmasking my autism* [Film]. BBC One. www.bbc.co.uk/programmes/m001k31t.

42. BBC. (2023, March 23). *Fi's journey to understanding her anorexia and autism* [Video]. YouTube. www.youtube.com/watch?v=wHQWYZ0JlZs.

43. Bourne, L., Bryant-Waugh, R., Cook, J., & Mandy, W. (2020). Avoidant/restrictive food intake disorder: A systematic scoping review of the current literature. *Psychiatry Research, 288*, 112961.

44. Koomar, T., Thomas, T. R., Pottschmidt, N. R., Lutter, M., & Michaelson, J. J. (2021). Estimating the prevalence and genetic risk mechanisms of ARFID in a large autism cohort. *Frontiers in Psychiatry, 12*, 668297.

45. Brede, J., Babb, C., Jones, C., Elliott, M., Zanker, C., Tchanturia, K., Serpell, L., Fox, J., & Mandy, W. (2020). 'For me, the anorexia is just a symptom, and the cause is the autism': Investigating restrictive eating disorders in autistic women. *Journal of Autism and Developmental Disorders, 50*(12), 4280–96.

46. So, P., Wierdsma, A. I., van Boeijen, C., Vermeiren, R. R., & Mulder,

N. C. (2021). Gender differences between adolescents with autism in emergency psychiatry. *Autism, 25*(8), 2331–40.

47. Steenfeldt-Kristensen, C., Jones, C. A., & Richards, C. (2020). The prevalence of self-injurious behaviour in autism: A meta-analytic study. *Journal of Autism and Developmental Disorders, 50*(11), 3857–73.

48. Farkas, B. F., Takacs, Z. K., Kollárovics, N., &Balázs, J. (2023, July 24). The prevalence of self-injury in adolescence: A systematic review and meta-analysis. *European Child & Adolescent Psychiatry*.

49. Blanchard, A., Chihuri, S., DiGuiseppi, C. G., & Li, G. (2021). Risk of self-harm in children and adults with autism spectrum disorder: A systematic review and meta-analysis. *JAMA Network Open, 4*(10), e2130272-e2130272.

50. Duerden, E. G., Oatley, H. K., Mak-Fan, K. M., McGrath, P. A., Taylor, M. J., Szatmari, P., & Roberts, S. W. (2012). Risk factors associated with self-injurious behaviors in children and adolescents with autism spectrum disorders. *Journal of Autism and Developmental Disorders, 42*(11), 2460–70; Steenfeldt-Kristensen, C., Jones, C. A., & Richards, C. (2020). The prevalence of self-injurious behaviour in autism: A meta-analytic study. *Journal of Autism and Developmental Disorders, 50*(11), 3857–73.

51. Cummings, L. R., Mattfeld, A. T., Pettit, J. W., & McMakin, D. L. (2021). Viewing nonsuicidal self-injury in adolescence through a developmental neuroscience lens: The impact of neural sensitivity to socioaffective pain and reward. *Clinical Psychological Science, 9*(5), 767–90.

52. Laye-Gindhu, A., & Schonert-Reichl, K. A. (2005). Nonsuicidal self-harm among community adolescents: Understanding the 'whats' and 'whys' of self-harm. *Journal of Youth and Adolescence, 34*, 447–57.

53. Bargiela, S., Steward, R., & Mandy, W. (2016). The experiences of late-diagnosed women with autism spectrum conditions: An investigation of the female autism phenotype. *Journal of Autism and Developmental Disorders, 46*(10), 3281–94.

54. Zucker, K. J., & Lawrence, A. A. (2009). Epidemiology of gender identity disorder: Recommendations for the *Standards of Care* of the World Professional Association for Transgender Health. *International Journal of Transgenderism, 11*(1), 8–18; Zucker, K. J. (2017). Epidemiology of gender dysphoria and transgender identity. *Sexual Health, 14*(5), 404–11.

55. Van Der Miesen, A. I. R., Hurley, H., & De Vries, A. L. C. (2018). Gender dysphoria and autism spectrum disorder: A narrative review. *Gender Dysphoria and Gender Incongruence*, 82–92; Glidden, D., Bouman, W. P., Jones, B. A., & Arcelus, J. (2016). Gender dysphoria and autism spectrum disorder: A systematic review of the literature. *Sexual Medicine Reviews, 4*(1), 3–14; Strang, J. F., Meagher, H., Kenworthy, L., de Vries, A. L. C., Menvielle, E., Leibowitz, S., et al. (2018). Initial clinical guidelines for co-occurring autism spectrum

disorder and gender dysphoria or incongruence in adolescents. *Journal of Clinical Child & Adolescent Psychology, 47*(1), 105–15.

56. de Vries, A. L. C., Noens, I. L. J., Cohen-Kettenis, P. T., van Berckelaer-Onnes, I. A., & Doreleijers, T. A. (2010). Autism spectrum disorders in gender dysphoric children and adolescents. *Journal of Autism and Developmental Disorders, 40*(8), 930–6; Pasterski, V., Gilligan, L., & Curtis, R. (2014). Traits of autism spectrum disorders in adults with gender dysphoria. *Archives of Sexual Behavior, 43*(2), 387–93.

57. Warrier, V., Greenberg, D. M., Weir, E., Buckingham, C., Smith, P., Lai, M.-C., Allison, C., & Baron-Cohen, S. (2020). Elevated rates of autism, other neurodevelopmental and psychiatric diagnoses, and autistic traits in transgender and gender-diverse individuals. *Nature Communications, 11*(1), 3959; Stagg, S. D., & Vincent, J. (2019). Autistic traits in individuals self-defining as transgender or nonbinary. *European Psychiatry, 61*, 17–22.

58. Cooper, K., Smith, L. G. E., & Russell, A. J. (2018). Gender identity in autism: Sex differences in social affiliation with gender groups. *Journal of Autism and Developmental Disorders, 48*(12), 3995–4006.

59. Brunissen, L., Rapoport, E., Chawarska, K., & Adesman, A. (2021). Sex differences in gender-diverse expressions and identities among youth with autism spectrum disorder. *Autism Research, 14*(1), 143–55; Kaltiala-Heino, R., Sumia, M., Työläjärvi, M., & Lindberg, N. (2015). Two years of gender identity service for minors: Overrepresentation of natal girls with severe problems in adolescent development. *Child and Adolescent Psychiatry and Mental Health, 9*, 1–9.

60. Pasterski, V., Zucker, K. J., Hindmarsh, P. C., Hughes, I. A., Acerini, C., Spencer, D., Neufeld, S., & Hines, M. (2015). Increased cross-gender identification independent of gender role behavior in girls with congenital adrenal hyperplasia: Results from a standardized assessment of 4- to 11-year-old children. *Archives of Sexual Behavior, 44*(5), 1363–75.

61. Moore, I., Morgan, G., Welham, A., & Russell, G. (2022). The intersection of autism and gender in the negotiation of identity: A systematic review and metasynthesis. *Feminism & Psychology, 32*(4), 421–42.

62. Strang, J. F., Powers, M. D., Knauss, M., Sibarium, E., Leibowitz, S. F., Kenworthy, L., Sadikova, E., Wyss, S., Willing, L., Caplan, R., and Pervez, N. (2018). "They thought it was an obsession": Trajectories and perspectives of autistic transgender and gender-diverse adolescents. *Journal of Autism and Developmental Disorders, 48*(12), 4039–55.

63. Turban, J. L., & van Schalkwyk, G. I. (2018). 'Gender dysphoria' and autism spectrum disorder: Is the link real? *Journal of the American Academy of Child & Adolescent Psychiatry, 57*(1), 8–9.

64. Strang, J. F., McClellan, L. S., Li, S., Jack, A. E., Wallace, G. L., McQuaid, G. A., Kenworthy, L., Anthony, L. G., Lai, M.-C., Pelphrey, K. A., Thalberg,

A. E., et al. (2023). The autism spectrum among transgender youth: Default mode functional connectivity. *Cerebral Cortex, 33*(11), 6633–47.

65. Horwitz, E., Vos, M., De Bildt, A., Greaves-Lord, K., Rommelse, N., Schoevers, R., & Hartman, C. (2023). Sex differences in the course of autistic and co-occurring psychopathological symptoms in adolescents with and without autism spectrum disorder. *Autism, 27*(6), 1716–29.

66. Gillberg, C. (1983). Are autism and anorexia nervosa related? *British Journal of Psychiatry, 142*(4), 428; Gillberg, C. (1985). Autism and anorexia nervosa: Related conditions? *Nordisk Psykiatrisk Tidsskrift*, 39(4), 307–12.

CONCLUSION. ASKING BETTER QUESTIONS, GETTING BETTER ANSWERS

1. Pellicano, E., & den Houting, J. (2022). Annual research review: Shifting from 'normal science' to neurodiversity in autism science. *Journal of Child Psychology and Psychiatry, 63*(4), 381–96; Pellicano, E., Lawson, W., Hall, G., Mahony, J., Lilley, R., Heyworth, M., Clapham, H., & Yudell, M. (2022). 'I knew she'd get it, and get me': Participants' perspectives of a participatory autism research project. *Autism in Adulthood, 4*(2), 120–9.

2. Patel, S. *30 sensory icks: A checklist for autistic and neurodivergent people*. Thinking Person's Guide to Autism. https://thinkingautismguide.com/2024/02/30-sensory-icks-a-checklist-for-autistic-and-neurodivergent-people.html.

3. Harrop, C., Tomaszewski, B., Putnam, O., Klein, C., Lamarche, E., & Klinger, L. (2024). Are the diagnostic rates of autistic females increasing? An examination of state-wide trends. *Journal of Child Psychology and Psychiatry, 65*(7), 973–83.

4. Tan, C. D. (2018). 'I'm a normal autistic person, not an abnormal neurotypical': Autism spectrum disorder diagnosis as biographical illumination. *Social Science & Medicine, 197*, 161–7.

5. Groen, Y., Ebert, W. M., Dittner, F. M., Stapert, A. F., Henning, D., Greaves-Lord, K., Davids, R. C. D., Castelein, S., Baron-Cohen, S., Allison, C., Van Balkom, I. D. C., & Piening, S. (2023). Measuring the autistic women's experience (AWE). *International Journal of Environmental Research and Public Health, 20*(24), 7148.

6. Clarke, E., Hull, L., Loomes, R., McCormick, C. E. B., Sheinkopf, S. J., & Mandy, W. (2021). Assessing gender differences in autism spectrum disorder using the Gendered Autism Behavioral Scale (GABS): An exploratory study. *Research in Autism Spectrum Disorders, 88*, 101844.

7. Baron-Cohen, S. (1997). *Mindblindness: An essay on autism and theory of mind*. MIT Press; Frith, U. (2003). *Autism: Explaining the enigma* (2nd ed.). Blackwell Publishing.

8. Rippon, G. (2024). Differently different? A commentary on the emerging social cognitive neuroscience of female autism. *Biology of Sex Differences, 15*(1), 49.

9. Criado Perez, C. (2019). *Invisible women: Data bias in a world designed for men*. Vintage.

10. Whipple, T. (2016, November 29). Sexism fears hamper brain research. *The Times*. www.thetimes.com/uk/science/article/sexism-fears-hamper-brain-research-rx6w39gbw.

11. Gillis-Buck, E., & Richardson, S. S. (2014). Autism as a biomedical platform for sex differences research. *BioSocieties, 9*(3), 262–83; Goldman, S. (2013). Opinion: Sex, gender and the diagnosis of autism – A biosocial view of the male preponderance. *Research in Autism Spectrum Disorders, 7*(6), 675–9.

12. Lai, M.-C., Lombardo, M. V., Suckling, J., Ruigrok, A. N. V., Chakrabarti, B., Ecker, C., Deoni, S. C. L., Craig, M. C., Murphy, D. G. M., Bullmore, E. T., & MRC AIMS Consortium (2013). Biological sex affects the neurobiology of autism. *Brain, 136*(9), 2799–2815.

13. Lai, M.-C., Lombardo, M. V., Chakrabarti, B., Ruigrok, A. N. V., Bullmore, E. T., Suckling, J., Auyeung, B., Happé, F., Szatmari, P., & Baron-Cohen, S. (2019). Neural self-representation in autistic women and association with 'compensatory camouflaging'. *Autism, 23*(5), 1210–23.

14. Floris, D. L., Peng, H., Warrier, V., Lombardo, M. V., Pretzsch, C. M., Moreau, C., Tsompanidis, A., Gong, W., Mennes, M., Llera, A., van Rooij, D., et al. (2023). The link between autism and sex-related neuroanatomy, and associated cognition and gene expression. *American Journal of Psychiatry, 180*(1), 50–64; Nogay, H. S., & Adeli, H. (2020). Machine learning (ML) for the diagnosis of autism spectrum disorder (ASD) using brain imaging. *Reviews in the Neurosciences, 31*(8), 825–41; Supekar, K., de Los Angeles, C., Ryali, S., Cao, K., Ma, T., & Menon, V. (2022). Deep learning identifies robust gender differences in functional brain organization and their dissociable links to clinical symptoms in autism. *British Journal of Psychiatry, 220*(4), 202–9.

15. Levy, Y. (2021). Commentary: Time to reconceptualize ASD? Comments on Happe and Frith (2020) and Sonuga-Barke (2020). *Journal of Child Psychology and Psychiatry, 62*(8), 1042–4; Lombardo, M. V., & Mandelli, V. (2022). Rethinking our concepts and assumptions about autism. *Frontiers in Psychiatry, 13*, 903489.

16. Müller, R.-A., & Fishman, I. (2018). Brain connectivity and neuroimaging of social networks in autism. *Trends in Cognitive Sciences, 22*(12), 1103–16.

17. Baron-Cohen, S. (2018, May 4). *Is it time to give up on a single diagnostic label for autism? Scientific American* blog. www.scientificamerican.com/blog/observations/is-it-time-to-give-up-on-a-single-diagnostic-label-for-autism.

18. Carpenter, B., Happé, F., & Egerton, J. (Eds.). (2019). *Girls and autism: Educational, family and personal perspectives*. Routledge.

19. TED. (2020, June 11). *A gendered world makes a gendered brain | Gina Rippon | TEDxCardiff* [Video]. YouTube. www.youtube.com/watch?v=2s1hrHppl5E.

20. Rippon, G. (2023). Mind the gender gap: The social neuroscience of belonging. *Frontiers in Human Neuroscience, 17,* 1094830.

21. Shansky, R. M., & Murphy, A. Z. (2021). Considering sex as a biological variable will require a global shift in science culture. *Nature Neuroscience, 24,* 457–64.

22. Nielsen, M. W., Stefanick, M. L., Peragine, D., Neilands, T. B., Ioannidis, J. P. A., Pilote, L., Prochaska, J. J., Cullen, M. R., Einstein, G., Klinge, I., LeBlanc, H., Paik, H. Y., & Schiebinger, L. (2021). Gender-related variables for health research. *Biology of Sex Differences, 12,* 1–16; Eliot, L., Beery, A. K., Jacobs, E. G., LeBlanc, H. F., Maney, D. L., & McCarthy, M. M. (2023). Why and how to account for sex and gender in brain and behavioral research. *Journal of Neuroscience, 43*(37), 6344–56.

23. Rippon, G. (2023). Mind the gender gap: The social neuroscience of belonging. *Frontiers in Human Neuroscience, 17,* 1094830.

24. The Fawcett Society. (2020, December). *Unlimited potential – The final report of the commission on gender stereotypes in early childhood.* www.fawcettsociety.org.uk/unlimited-potential-the-final-report-of-the-commission-on-gender-stereotypes-in-early-childhood; Geena Davis Institute. *LEGO ready for girls creativity study.* https://geenadavisinstitute.org/research/lego-ready-for-girls-creativity-study.

25. Milton, D., Gurbuz, E., & López, B. (2022). The 'double empathy problem': Ten years on. *Autism, 26*(8), 1901–3.

26. Edwards, C., Love, A. M. A., Jones, S. C., Cai, R. Y., Nguyen, B. T. H., & Gibbs, V. (2024). 'Most people have no idea what autism is': Unpacking autism disclosure using social media analysis. *Autism, 28*(5), 1107–19.

27. Mandy, W. (2019). Social camouflaging in autism: Is it time to lose the mask? *Autism, 23*(8), 1879–81.

28. Cook, J., Hull, L., & Mandy, W. (2024). Improving diagnostic procedures in autism for girls and women: A narrative review. *Neuropsychiatric Disease and Treatment, 20,* 505–14; Lai, M.-C., Amestoy, A., Bishop, S., Brown, H. M., Onaiwu, M. G., Halladay, A., Harrop, C., Hotez, E., Huerta, M., Kelly, A., Miller, D., et al. (2023). Improving autism identification and support for individuals assigned female at birth: Clinical suggestions and research priorities. *The Lancet Child & Adolescent Health, 7*(12), 897–908.

INDEX